MW01292675

The COMPLETE GUIDE to EATING the
PROTEIN to LOSE FAT, GAIN MUSCLE,

The
PROTEIN PACING DIET

Backed by Real Human Nutrition and Applied Physiology Research Studies!

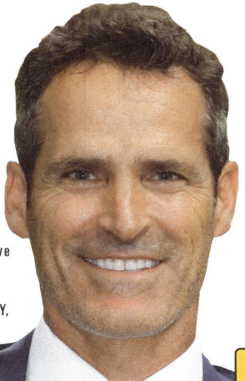

"You can finally achieve
OPTIMAL HEALTH
and FITNESS."

—STEPHEN M.R. COVEY,
From the Foreword

**PRISE®
App Included**

Dr. PAUL J. ARCIERO

Outskirts Press, Inc.
http://www.outskirtspress.com

Paperback ISBN: 978-1-4787-9947-4
Hardback ISBN: 978-1-4787-9948-1

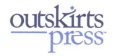

Table of Contents

Part Three
Dr. Paul's PRISE Life Protocol Revealed

Time to RISE Up! (Fitness Is...LIFE...)

P-PROTEIN PACING
R-RESISTANCE
I-INTERVAL
S-STRETCHING
E-ENDURANCE

Part Four
The Archer Behind the PRISE

Praise for Dr. Paul

"I've known Dr. Paul since 2009. Then, at age 55, I began a march from a Lazy-Boy-Chair lifestyle to a 2011 gold-medal winning, National Cycling Championship podium. In two short years, Dr. Paul helped me achieve what seemed to everyone around me to be the impossible. By following his nutrition, exercise and health protocols, I leapfrogged competitors who'd been diligently training for decades. Best of all, I returned to vibrant health after decades of sacrificing myself to the rigors and requirements of high-performing entrepreneurship and impactful business. At 57 years old, I only had one shot at a championship medal. I only have one life to live. I'm grateful I was wise enough to put both in Dr. Paul's capable hands."

Bill Watkins, world-class athlete, founder of
The Lions Pride, husband, father, adventurer

"Whether you are an elite athlete, weekend warrior, or an individual who is just trying to improve the quality of life through diet and exercise, this book belongs within arms reach of your exercise equipment and food preparation station. Dr. Paul, masterfully guides the reader through a maze of diets and exercise programs. Dr. Paul's writing style personally reaches out to you, to guide you in improving your performance. He navigates through current complex and sometimes conflicting research on nutrition and exercise and designs a comprehensive evidence based program with his passionate prose."

Gaetano J. Scuderi, MD, Certified Orthopedic Spine Surgeon,
Cytonics Corporation Founder, Clinical Assistant Professor,
Orothopedic and Spine Surgery, Stanford University

"Dr. Paul is transforming lives with 'The Protein Pacing Diet' because it shares innovative insights and strategies for enhancing your health. Get Excited because this book will truly empower you and your family. Remember, Your Health is Your Wealth."

Marlon Smith, Tony Robbins Global Youth Leadership Summit Trainer,
Contributing Author to International Best-Selling "Chicken Soup for the Soul"

"Dr. Paul's Protein Pacing and PRISE Protocol is a total game changer, helping people from all walks of life achieve optimal health and fitness. This book is a must read, and I believe will be instrumental in creating a health and fitness movement that we have not yet experienced in this century."

David T.S. Wood, Speaker, Trainer & Philanthropist

"Dr. Paul's Protein Pacing Diet eloquently combines his outstanding scientific acumen and passion for us all to lead fulfilling and meaningful lives by successfully optimizing human performance, health, and relationships. Paul's innate ability to care for, nurture, and develop relationships with others is clearly present here as he shares personal experiences of struggle, joy, sacrifice, and success that help us embrace the importance of the holistic and balanced nutrition and exercise principles that culminated in PRISE. Dr. Pauls Protein Pacing Diet truly embodies his life-long mission of guiding us to lives rich in love and joy."

Meghan Downs, PhD, NASA Johnson Space Center Exercise
Physiology and Performance Discipline Lead

"Paul Arciero is a gifted scientist, athlete, and exemplar for nutrition, health and fitness as he truly 'talks the talk and walks the walk'. The information he provides in 'Dr. Paul's Protein Pacing Diet' is germane to nutrition and fitness and will prove to be transformative for everyone disciplined to apply his scientifically proven principles into their lifestyles. A truly inspirational author and book."

Bradley C. Nindl, Ph.D., Director, Neuromuscular Research Laboratory/
Warrior Human Performance Research Center, University of Pittsburgh

"Dr Arciero's work and personality is eloquently captured in this book. This is his Sistine Chapel ceiling. He poured his soul writing this book with uncluttered, clear and much needed actionable advice. Read it, apply it and share this beautiful work. I have!"

Ara Suppiah MD, Emergency and Sports Medicine Physician,
2016/2018 US Ryder Cup Team Physician, Chief Medical Analyst for
NBC Sports Golf Channel, Chief Medical Officer for Orreco US Operations

"I was fortunate to work with Dr. Paul in my journey training and competing in my 4th and 5th Olympic competitions in Short Track Speed Skating. Having once had aspirations of getting a Masters in Exercise Physiology, I appreciate the massive amounts of research, hard work and personal commitment Dr. Paul continues to pour into his work; as he did with me in our time together. Now, as a super busy mother of 4 boys — which only the Olympics could have prepared me for, I can say all the more how with busy schedules, Protein Pacing and the PRISE Life protocol answers all our needs to stay in shape. Dr. Paul helps us understand how our bodies work the most efficiently and keep us fit for what he calls this 'race of life.' Dr. Paul is a remarkable resource for the sports science community."

Amy Peterson, USA Short Track 5 time Olympian (1 silver medal, 2 bronze medals). Olympic Games: 1988 Calgary; 1992 Albertville; 1994 Lillehammer Olympics; 1998 Nagano; 2002 Salt Lake City where she was elected to carry the USA flag at the Opening Ceremony. In 2000-2001 she was ranked #9 in the World

"In todays' fast-paced world, there are many shortcuts to better health. Dr Paul Arciero's PRISE Life is truly the way to a healthy lifestyle, better performance and a happier life, and like most things in life, it's not always easy, but it's correct. Wish I had seen this 30 years ago!"

Brad Faxon, FOX Sports Golf Analyst, 8 time PGA Champion, Top 20 World Golf Ranking, 2 time Ryder Cup Player

"Dr. Paul's 'Protein Pacing Diet and PRISE Life' book is a must read for anyone striving for optimal health, fitness and peak performance. I have been present at many of Dr. Paul's talks on Protein Pacing and was thoroughly excited to read his book on such a fascinating and progressive concept. He truly lives the life as a leading scientist, keynote, consultant, and athlete!"

Chris Algieri, M.S., CISSN, Former World Boxing Champion, 2x World Kickboxing Champion, Performance Nutrition Specialist

Dedication

To Grandpa John Petrillo, Grandma Deedie Arciero, Donald Vincent Arciero, and Jane Barbara (Petrillo) Arciero

This book is dedicated to you, my devoted research "subjects," clients, students, and ever-growing group of supporters now reaching into the millions. It seems that destiny called me well before I arrived at the idea to write this book, but it is clear now that everything links back to what you have graciously taught me along the way.

While I continue to work diligently to find different ways to provide you with the most successful, safest, and easiest lifestyle strategies, know that I want to offer the very best to you. I want you to become so inspired, motivated, and successful that you are driven to share this recipe to living your *best* life with others. What has become a well-documented and scientifically proven roadmap (Protein Pacing and the PRISE Life) to achieving optimal health and peak performance is now yours to finally attain—and it is all thanks to your devotion in helping me commit to the scientific process.

Remember, we all have deficits; perhaps we have even been told we are "defective." Don't listen. Not only is there a special path for you but there is one that brings you success, optimal health, and peak performance. Above all, know that I am devoted to you finding a deep love of yourself, a gift that in return will honor you with a truly fulfilling and meaningful life—the kind that I have been so blessed to find.

Acknowledgments

Although I have dedicated my professional career to being a nutrition and applied physiology research scientist, international media personality and keynote speaker, college professor, coach, and consultant, I have always placed my relationship with others as the most meaningful and fulfilling blessing of what I do. For me, developing a nurturing and caring environment from which I conduct my research, teach my students, coach my athletes, mentor and guide my clients, work alongside colleagues, and motivate my audiences has been at the core of everything I do. It is this atmosphere that has created a rock-solid foundation for my Protein Pacing and PRISE Life strategies to assure that they survive "the test of time" and serve millions more well into the future.

I am eternally grateful for the love and support of my family and friends who always believe in me, my passions, and my dedication to helping others live a life of optimal health and peak performance.

My mother, Jane Barbara (Petrillo) Arciero, (a vibrant and active nurturer— "The eighty-four-year-old hiking grandma") who along with my father, Donald Vincent Arciero, ("Big D," your spirit lives on forever for living every day with humility and grace), you were at the forefront of living a life of optimal health and peak performance. You inspired my earliest entry into the field of nutrition, fitness, and health and created my *essence* of being.

My grandfather, John Petrillo, and grandmother, Edith (Deedie) Dean Arciero. You gave me constant love and always believed in me when I didn't always believe in myself. Your legacies live on in me and my family every day.

My older brother, John. You have always been a constant source of support, confidence, and mentoring in everything I have done in life. Thank you for always believing that my *message* for optimal health and peak performance was going to be the leading voice.

My amazing brothers Chris, Peter, and Matt, and sisters Donna and Jackie. Combined, you created the most wonderful gift of family, love, and support. Each of you, in your own unique and powerful way, have blessed my life beyond words.

My best friend and beautiful wife, Karen. Thank you for always support-ing me and believing in me. You have been by my side always providing the level-headed voice of reason I needed to stay on track all while encouraging my creativity. I'm grateful for your excellent feedback on this book, with everything from organization, to putting my thoughts into easily understood words, to ad-vice with citations. Your constant encouragement keeps me strong. You remain the greatest source of my *essence, mission* (passion), *message*, and *blessing*.

My three amazing and gifted sons Nicholas, Noah, and Aidan. You are the life source of my *mission*, energy, and motivation. You surpass me in every way of existence, matched only by the love we have for each other.

Each of these incredible people have been the driving force behind Dr. Paul's PRISE Life, including Protein Pacing and the primary reason it has become and will remain the most successful path to optimal health and peak performance. I have been truly blessed with a remarkable team of supporters; therefore, this book and its discoveries are as much yours as they are mine.

I love each one of you with all my heart, mind, and soul.

Special Thanks

This book started as a work in progress beginning when I was a young boy searching for meaning and a path in life. Several challenging and early-life transforming events questioned my self-worth and identity, but nurturing grandparents, parents, and siblings revealed their unconditional love and belief in me. Good or bad, life experiences are the *essence* of who I am today. Soon after, I witnessed some of these same loved ones becoming ill or diseased, and this deeply touched my inner soul and quickly stoked the flame of my passion and eventual *mission* in life—that being to help others live a life of optimal health and peak performance.

For the past thirty years in scientific research (and almost fifty years "personal experience" in nutrition, health, and fitness), this book has taken form as I began my career as a nutrition and applied physiology college professor and scientist, as well as a performance coach, mentor, scientific advisory board member, and leading worldwide expert/spokesperson in nutrition, fitness, and health. These roles have provided me an incredible platform to spread my *message*, and I am grateful and humbled for each opportunity I'm provided.

I owe much of my inspiration to finally complete this book to my loving family and friends, the thousands of students in my classes and labs, the athletes I've coached, the hundreds of research study participants, brilliant colleagues, and the millions of people my research, teaching, mentoring, and coaching has influenced over the years.

A special thanks to my dear friend and exceptional health coach and journalist, Jessica Cassity for the initial brainstorming and jumpstart to collecting my thoughts and putting them to paper. It was because of their persistent and constant encouragement of me to put into words and onto paper all of my healthy lifestyle strategies of Protein Pacing and PRISE I was finally able to "follow through" and share with all of you my ultimate *blessing* of this book! I am grateful for their faith and belief in me as an evangelist and change agent to serve as their motivation for a "life-changing experience" leading to optimal health and peak performance.

It is now my honor to thank and introduce Stephen M.R. Covey, the great inspirational and motivational author and speaker who has been kind enough to share his thoughts on this book and the process. Having his personal endorsement means everything to me.

Foreword

Principles.

Universal truths.

Enduring foundations on which the world operates.

My late father, Dr. Stephen R. Covey, studied, practiced, and taught principles of leadership and effectiveness throughout his life. I've followed his example in seeking to deeply understand and share the lasting principles upon which trusting relationships, organizations, and societies are built and prosper.

Now Dr. Paul Arciero has done the same with the enduring principles that ensure human health, fitness, and performance. What a wonderful contribution this is!

I'll never forget the day I met Dr. Paul. We were both speaking at a conference several years ago when we first conversed and then later that day we found ourselves at the airport headed to our next destinations where we had another discussion. I found Paul to be a credible and trusted source for the principles and practices of health and fitness, and equally important, a sincere and genuine individual driven by a mission in life to help people optimize their health and happiness.

In Western societies, we are struggling with epidemic levels of obesity, diabetes, heart disease, cancers, and many new lifestyle-related diseases. They are rapidly increasing because people are unaware, misinformed, or ignoring the basic principles of wise eating, exercise, and energy management. That's where Dr. Paul's work comes in. Backed by scientific data and peer-reviewed research, Dr. Paul lays out the principles that underlie health and fitness in a way that challenges our age-old assumptions and shifts our paradigms.

As you study this marvelous book, you will gain greater understanding, and motivation to practice, the principles of health and vitality that Paul calls the PRISE Protocol. Fad diets and body-punishing exercise regimes are much like the get-rich-quick, pop psychology advice you see in hundreds of books and websites. By contrast, the principles that undergird PRISE are sound, based on peer-reviewed research, then published in credible scientific journals. This is not a "get-fit-quick" solution. It's a solid, beneficial program of resistance, high-intensity interval, stretching, and endurance training, proper eating, and sleep that, if followed, will deliver on its promise.

For example, Dr. Paul breaks ground on what pacing your protein really means—how he created it, how the timing of what you eat is critical, and how much of what types of food you eat can literally change your life. He teaches us the value of high-quality nourishment and fitness training to improve energy metabolism, body composition, glucose tolerance, and lessening of cardiovascular disease risk by losing adipose tissue (especially belly fat) and how exactly to gain more control over our body and health.

But don't worry, with the empirical data to back up his PRISE Life protocol, Dr. Paul makes this an easy-to-read book, reminding us about macros (those proteins, fats, and carbohydrates), and then simplifies everything with easy-to-follow charts. You can finally achieve the optimal health and fitness you have always dreamed about and might even be able to push yourself to peak performance levels that you had long given up on.

This is a very current and important piece of work. Dr. Paul shows that although a healthy lifestyle takes commitment, nutrition and exercise don't need to be as complicated as we are being led by the hype to believe. Of course, a healthy lifestyle incorporates exercise, but it is amazing how much easier movement is when we feel good or don't have such extreme time and energy-expending hurdles to overcome to demotivate us. He demonstrates how energy is our life's force and how ultimately we want the same thing—health and longevity to spend quality time doing what we love with and for our loved ones. For me, this works for us folks with busy work schedules, all the way to the Olympians or star athletes. Dr. Paul knows—he was a tennis champion himself and shares his struggles and journeys in a wonderful heartfelt chapter.

I've validated these principles myself through years of struggling with my weight fluctuating up and down (mostly up) as I've attempted to manage constant global travel, meals on the run, and a jam-packed schedule as an executive and now as a professional speaker and author. Even though I have a discipline of exercising at least thirty minutes every day, I've learned several new strategies and approaches in this book that I'm confident will take me to the next level of fitness and performance.

Perhaps what has been most inspirational to me in Paul's book is his explanation of who trusted him. While it's not a primary emphasis in the Protein Pacing Diet, it's the primary driver of how this work came to be. I loved reading how he found his voice as a young person and pursued that passion through his academic studies, as a competitive athlete, and as a gifted human being. And how did he find his voice? By the encouragement and support of loved ones, especially "Grandma Deedie," "Grandpa," "Big D," his dad, and his mother, the "84-year-old hiking grandmother." I love to hear, collect, and share the stories of how people respond when they're trusted, and I believe you will be inspired as you read Paul's and enjoy the results from applying the teachings of this book.

Thank you, Paul, for your wonderful work and for the pleasure it gives me to see how you have focused on principles in the health and fitness dimension, much like my father and I have focused on principles in the human and organizational effectiveness dimension. Seeing a parallel focus around universal principles is what continues to make my life infinitely rewarding.

I look forward to our next "chance" encounter on the speaking circuit or even at an airport!

Stephen M. R. Covey, Author of *The New York Times*
and #1 *Wall Street Journal* best-selling book, *The Speed of Trust,*
Former President & CEO of Covey Leadership Center

Introduction

Let me begin this book by sharing that I am going to take you on a journey—a journey about life and what a healthy lifestyle really means. All of us have a journey, and this is mine. My goal is to help you live your journey healthier and with better nutrition, fitness, and performance. This is not just a regular diet and fitness book like the handfuls that seem to come out monthly, connected to e-books, e-mails, newsletters, monthly fees, and the latest and greatest ways to lose weight or gain muscle. This book is the culmination of a deep belief that science mimics the perfection of nature and that if we follow its "rules," the way we were originally created (which may be simpler than we are led to believe), we can all achieve optimal health and fitness, and even longevity.

I understand this is a bold statement in a world where we want things quick and we want things cheap. I am here to tell you that a bunch of flimsy theories thrown together, that will solve only a portion of the population's problems, is no solution at all. I am also here to tell you that after thirty years of research as a scientist and breaking down all these up-and-coming—some fly-by-night—ideas, there is an actual roadmap, protocol, *recipe* in fact, *key*, to finding and achieving health. It is no longer a mystery, and it absolutely does not have to cost you a fortune. Throughout this book, I share the science behind my PRISE Life protocol, including my discovery of Protein Pacing, providing sources to peer reviewed material with proven science to establish even further credibility as to how the process works. Finally, I guide you through the simple and easy steps that evolved from my own personal dilemma of needing a program that worked in our stressful world where we find ourselves short of time. You will hear some stories that fueled my passion to get others healthy so you too can "Keep Your Eyes on the PRISE" and finally claim the ultimate weight and longevity you deserve. I introduce you to the application of Protein Pacing and the PRISE Protocol so you can seamlessly and synergistically incorporate these into your own life to help give you the best results you've ever seen. But, please keep in mind, I will have two additional books and the PRISE App coming out soon on how to perform each of the components of PRISE in much greater detail. Please visit www.paularciero.com, www.proteinpacing.com, and www.priseprotocol. com often to join our PRISE and Protein Pacing community.

This book is a journey because I share with you how this discovery came about and how you, too, can implement it to change your life. With my research devoted to human performance, nutrition, and applied physiology, as well as neuropsychology and cognitive development, I have happened upon some of the most fascinating results as to how the human body functions the best, the way nature intended it to be without overexertion, dehydration, crazy 500-calorie-a-day diets, injections, steroids, medications, bypass surgeries, sugar-packed meal replacement powders and bars, stimulants, deprivation, overanalyzing, and the list goes on.

I am going to share with you ground-breaking studies from the relatively new and exciting fields of human performance, nutrition, neuroscience, and applied physiology. According to the American College of Sport Medicine (ACSM), the leading and most respected authority on sports medicine and related fields, it states in the nutrition science guidelines that, "Nutrition for sport is the provision of essential nutrients, including fuels and fluids, to provide energy for training, competition, recovery, and general health and wellness. The intake versus expenditure of these essential nutrients will be called energy balance. Optimum performance is promoted by adequate energy intake."[1] This is exactly what I am doing when I am researching what foods to eat when, in what quantity, how much fluid is needed, and how this pertains to either recovery or greater wellness in my subjects. We need energy to live, and there is an actual method to getting the proper nutrition to support the human body.

As for achieving health, isn't the core of life all about the nutrition part of eating right, getting the proper fluids into the body, and then exercising properly? I know, this may make some people cringe or complain, but the common held belief to a healthy lifestyle is you must eat less and exercise more. But my message is nearly the *opposite* of this ... I am actually going to show you a way to eat more high-quality foods and pay less attention to the quantity of food you eat and, then, how to exercise smarter not harder and longer. So, hold on, hold on, I will get there!

---

1   "Selected Issues for Nutrition and the Athlete: Medicine & Science in Sports & Exercise." LWW. Accessed February 2, 2018. https://journals.lww.com/acsm-msse/Fulltext/2013/12000/Selected_Issues_ for_Nutrition_and_the_Athlete_A.21.aspx.

One creative description defined exercise science and applied physiology as "the study of the acute responses and chronic adaptations to a wide range of nutrition supplementation and exercise conditions."[2] It's interesting to note that as the field has developed, *supplementation* and *exercise* are words and concepts being joined together more often. The wording is interesting because the conflict of response then adaptation reminds me of life. Isn't life about constantly having acute responses to situations, and aren't we chronically adapting to new or different circumstances? Something to think about!

For the portion of my job that is defined as an applied physiologist, I study physiology and the ways in which it impacts human health and performance. Specifically, I'm interested in the interaction between environmental factors, nutrition, exercise, and disease on human function, as well as the physiological mechanisms regulating human health and performance. I work to understand how to reverse disease progression and how to encourage peak physical performance, always working from the level the person is currently at, to safely increase their results. Again, isn't this what we do in life as we use our bodies as science experiments? Aren't we always researching and seeking ways that, with proper nutrition and exercise, we can work to attain optimal health, perhaps even sustained peak performance, and reverse disease all for the goal of living a long and healthy life? Or, in simpler terms, aren't we just working to look and feel better? One of the themes I've grown to embrace is "it's not how fast you start, but how long you last." In other words, consistency wins every time. This is what PRISE with Protein Pacing is all about.

I know that in the past I've been the scientist hidden in the lab, but now I am here to *share* my research with you. That's my current stage. Because life, in the end, is lived in stages, and each stage leads us through a journey, and each journey can lead to bettering human kind or hindering the future of our planet and our lives. Which path do you choose? I'm hoping that with the information I share with you in this book, you will find the motivation to throw away all those crazy temporary diet ideas and exercise fads and follow my roadmap of the PRISE Protocol with Protein Pacing and choose optimal health and peak performance!

---

2   "Definition." American Society of Exercise Physiologists. Accessed December 18, 2017. https://www. asep.org/about-asep/definition/.

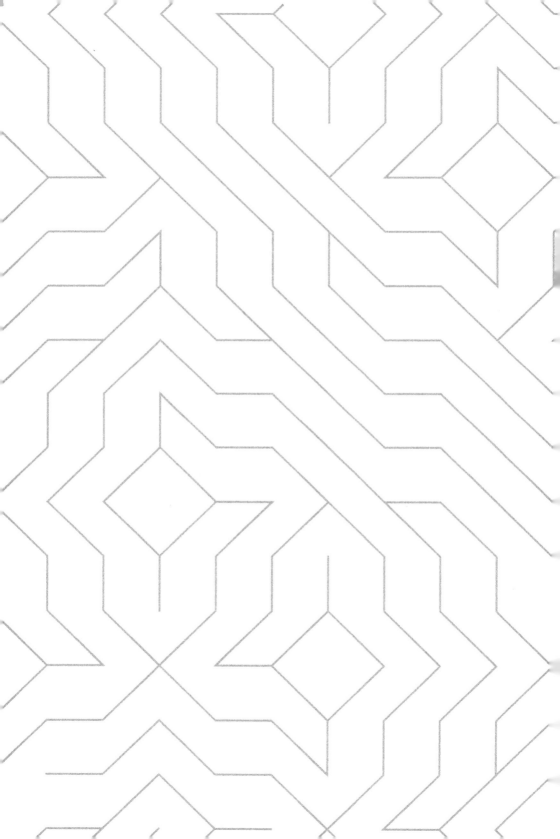

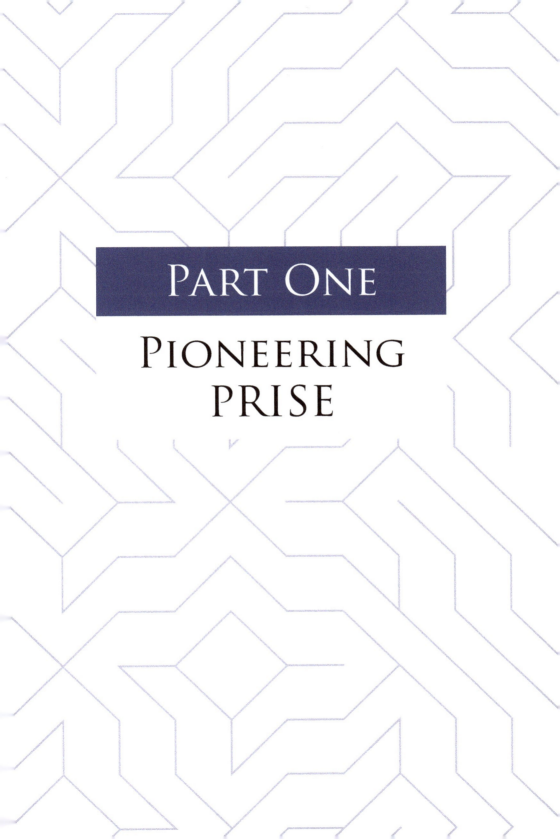

PART ONE

PIONEERING
PRISE

1

The Journey

Life is what happens to you while you are busy making other plans.
—John Lennon

As I said in the introduction, I am going to take you on a journey, a "revealing" in a sense and then a true discovery that I am excited to share as it makes its way around the world with your help. Like most discoveries, it didn't happen in a bubble, and it did take years of peeling the layers back to find the answer. But I don't want you to just walk away with another quick discovery. I want you to walk away with a willingness, a drive, and a desire to make a personal change for the better for you and for your loved ones. The reason being is that life can be hard, and we can all be fragile at times. If my life stories help you see that you are not the only person who has ever suffered, then perhaps the discoveries I have made will make sense and become the building blocks to a new and healthier life for all those you touch: I refer to this as "geometric growth" and the "force multiplier" or ripple effect, as some call it.

Before I get into all the specifics of my scientific breakthroughs, which are detailed in part 3, I want to share a little human psychology; because in the end we are mind, body, and spirit, and to live a balanced and healthy life, we need to take all this into account. Yes, I am a scientist, I believe in defined, explained, and rational scientifically proven data, but I am also a human being who does believe in the power of the mind and positive intention-based thinking. As I have evolved, I have come to embrace the spiritual components of life more and more. When combining all three, and as most top achievers or simply happy people will concur, you can finally reach your dreams.

Human development combines physical growth with the psychological cycle of life. Different ages and stages of our lives present us with different tasks to conquer.[3] With five and a half decades to my development emotionally, physically, and spiritually, I have discovered that I am living proof of this. I am finally in that odd position where I can look back past the ups and downs of my early years and start to make sense of this amazing journey or science experiment called life.

Without getting too complicated, when we are young, we are egocentric; we have the "magical thinking" of the seven- and eight-year-old. We focus on what everyone else is getting and what we are not getting. You may have had a healthy start to life with nurturing parents, or you may have had a difficult start, one wracked with deprivation and neglect, leaving you frustrated, upset, hurt, or even lost. You live a lot of your life in the pretend world to make up for the facets of nurturance you might not have received, or you spend your time dreaming of better things to come, because that's what we as humans do. Even if you were blessed with a wonderful and nurturing home life to start, you will spend time dreaming in this "imagination" mode. It could be of the day you win an Olympic Gold medal, become a famous actor, win a Nobel Peace prize, or simply have a healthy simple life; no matter our situations, this magical thinking stage helps to plan our future or work through life's lessons.

As you age, ego takes hold, and it may or may not have your best interest in mind. You start getting trapped in the real world of hard knocks, all while trying to bring mind, body, and spirit into harmony and balance. You find yourself conflicted between your need for immediate gratification, recognition, love, and acceptance and comparing yourself to others. The criticizing authoritarian in your mind jumps in. You either become an extrovert, the competitor, the one who is the best, and can be "seen," or you start to retreat into introversion. Introversion is where you find things to keep you occupied, often alone, so as to avoid others. This may simply be because you are just that uncomfortable around people, or you may have learned a defense mechanism—that conscious mental process built in to protect you. To protect your ego, you decide you want to avoid criticism, internal anxiety, or ostracism and thereby remain as "unseen" as possible. I can relate to this for sure!

No matter the psychological type you start to pattern, all human behaviors are shaped (some might say predetermined) by the size of family you come

---

3   "PsycNET," American Psychological Association, accessed January 8, 2018, http://psycnet.apa.org/record/1975-26412-001.

from, the positive or negative people around you, the levels of nurturance you receive, and the groups that you attach yourself to as you mature, whether it is the athletes, the intellectuals, the nerds, the cool ones, or whatever stereotype that exists today. You start discovering some of the nature-given strengths you were born with, whether good looks, a sense of humor, a strong athletic ability, or high intelligence, and you start to define who you want to become or "be"— as in career aspirations. But be forewarned; these gifts don't come free. Where one strength rules, there are many weaknesses just waiting to oppose. The conscious and subconscious are in constant struggle.

You start to juggle life and realize you need to decide what you are going to do with it. Perhaps go to college or become a top athlete, and in this dreaming, wishing, hoping, and working toward some goals or aspirations, you start to experience new thoughts and understandings. For example, this is much harder than I thought it would be. What was I thinking? However, with persistence and a few successes under your belt, you become cognizant of the fact that you might actually have a talent and might even be the master of your own destiny!

You start to know who you are. You start to define and determine who you are. It feels great. You are in charge!

Or, so you think.

Because just as you think you have that mastered, something steps in the way. Or as John Lennon says, "Life is what happens to you while you are busy making other plans."

With these few successes, and hopefully many more failures behind you, your life evolves. And for most people, we become less egocentric and start to crave deeper relationships and bonds. This has its good and bad sides because it encourages you to create new relationships, but as time goes on you find yourself, sadly, losing those you love either due to different belief systems or worse yet illness and death. I know, I've had that pain and it has changed my life.

No matter how much you think you are in control, your deeper underlying purpose and virtue and the cycle of life can't be ignored. You carry memories within you of all sorts, and you get molded and defined by each action and reaction. That is science. That is nature. That is faith and spirituality.

But you persevere again, and now it is your turn to start to teach others what you have learned yourself. You may start to have children of your own, or you may go into teaching or instructing, or a life of service, or you may decide that no, actually, you want none of that because you are on the top of your game and this is the time for you to shine. It is the constant roller coaster of growing pains of life and love and the dichotomies I refer to as the "karmic cul-de-sac"; disappointment and fulfillment; challenges and opportunities; failure and success... and failure, again, and next thing you know you are a professional, in your mid-fifties, just like me, and it feels as though life has just flown by. Of the many life lessons I've learned over the years, there is a need for failure, and in some cases massive failure! Because, ultimately, it's the experience of failure that provides us the momentum to swing in the other direction toward success. Never fear failure; instead, embrace it and use it to create inertia to move in the other direction toward huge success.

A weird convergence transpires: The lines or roads and crazy detours seem to make uncanny sense because they have led you to this exact moment. Well, that moment for me is what this book is all about.

As a scientist, I have carefully analyzed, written, studied, restudied, taught, and looked at data from all angles. I have spent my life trying to figure out why we humans react and act as we humans do. In my case, my passion has been through human nutrition and applied physiology. And although it started as a more egocentric need to be the best athlete I could, and to beat all others in competition whether it was hockey, tennis, triathlons, etc., there was an internal drive in me pushing to be the best.

I never really thought about it in this way, until I started giving speeches. Now I know this convergence was probably no "accident" at all.

Ironically, it is crazy when I personally look back and realize that my journey to optimal health and *peak* performance started as a first grader when my teachers wanted to "hold me back" to repeat the school year. I had no intellectual "peak" in sight—see irony and a hefty dose of "believed" failure. It then happened *again* in fifth grade when I was placed in "special" classes for remedial learners. More irony. To add to those painful failures, and being separated out from others, I also came from one of those large Italian families, seven children in total, and sure enough I was one of the middle ones you hear about—the kind that gets lost in the crowd. You can have a great family and still just be that one stuck in the middle. Therefore, my "formative years," as developmental psychologists call it, had events, situations, and interactions that were massive blows to my self-worth and self-esteem, and to this day they continue to influence my life in many ways.

Hold tight, though, because all was not lost. Although one door, the intellectual/academic future one, felt like it had slammed shut, another door, an appreciation for my physical health and desire to compete, began to open for me—more out of survival than anything else. This is the amazing story I have to tell.

On the coming pages I share with you how my experience as a young boy, who struggled terribly in school, found his life calling by learning; sometimes serendipitously, about the right type and amount of high-quality food and physical activity; sometimes by having a few fortunate role models who believed in me when I didn't believe in myself; and sometimes having those interventionists who taught me the value of appreciating the life-giving potential of nourishing the body with high-quality foods while implementing fitness and exercise. Eventually, the daily lessons of failure, trial and error, and rough times all converged. Whatever life had in mind, it eventually created the inertia and momentum I needed to develop resolve and a healthy dose of spiritual and emotional fulfillment combined with nutrition and smart/safe levels of exercise. In other words, *balance*. And although none of this came easy, it is the reason I am writing this book today.

I have learned that development, then balance, also applies to nutrition and is something I have researched more. The life cycle of plants is just as crucial as the psychological life cycle of humans and has so many things to teach us. I was lucky enough to have the "seed" of nutrition planted in me early—I tell my story more fully at the end of this book, but my mother taught me to nourish my body using what comes from the earth. It is her lessons that I share when I teach you to "eat dirty," play in the garden, and realize that true nourishment comes in many ways. Growing your own food source from the earth's soil is ultimately the greatest source of nourishment to keep our body healthy and functioning at the highest level. It's a topic I address along with nutrition facts, because our modern world is taking all the "life" out of us and the food we eat.

Mother Earth is, undoubtedly, still the prime nourisher, and if we focus on the quality of soil, replenishing enzymes, and restoring agriculture, as it was supposed to be without all the added chemicals and pesticides, replace what minerals have been robbed from us while focusing on high-quality (whole) foods and even supplements, we will become a healthier world. The garden teaches us everything we need to know in life: When to plant a seed, when and how much water is needed, getting necessary sunshine and when it's time to be in the shade, how to grow strong or rest, when to add extra nourishment when some quality is missing, when to remove bugs and when to add bugs. The whole cycle of human nutrition can be found in the seasons, in gardening, and the organisms. It is an environment that supports all life. Nurturing a living organism through its "life cycle" is physically and spiritually one of the most significant actions one can participate in. It's something I encourage everyone to try because there are deeply satisfying feelings when you bring food fresh from your garden right to your table. You will even find it bursting with so much flavor that you will probably wonder why you didn't try this sooner.

Although this book focuses more on the nutrition, fitness, and the optimal performance end, I want to take a moment to talk about *emotional* nurturance from food and exercise. Eating foods that contain all the vital and essential nutrients (vitamins, minerals, phytochemicals) that originate primarily from the earth or garden, or even today in reputable nature-based supplements and meal-replacement protein powders and bars, make us strong. Fake foods, which often lead to unhealthy cravings and addictions, make us weak. But by combining healthy nutrition with exercise and fitness routines, research has proven that a smart integration will net significant mood enhancement results. We all feel better, have more energy, and clearer thinking when we fuel our bodies with nutritious, healthy food. You hear about the "runner's high" and have probably experienced that exuberance after a really challenging, but fun, team sport, being active outdoors in nature, or a time you pushed yourself further than ever before. All these actions create endorphins, as well as other positive biochemical reactions, and in combination help your body support your mind. Positive thinking is so much easier when you feel good, right?

As a result, the stages of *my* life with the types of emotional, physical, spiritual, "nutrition," and at times "deprivation," as well as quantifiable research, have been invaluable as I have tried to make sense of achieving optimal health and peak performance. This is what ultimately inspired me to become a change leader and evangelist. I moved from that egocentric world of just wanting to figure out how to be the best athlete I could be and learned I actually liked helping others get there too, even more. This gave me a deeper sense of fulfillment and meaning.

This is what drives me today. To inspire others to embrace their health and take control of the daily lifestyle choices is what has pushed me to work so hard and want to take a risk not only to write this book but share the gifts given to me. The need to show others how to improve their overall health and fitness, with scientific proof to back it up, has consumed me, but it now makes sense. The result: My brain child (the program that has now become popularly referred to as Dr. Paul's PRISE Life Protocol, this overarching lifestyle program) was born. The execution of daily lifestyle strategies that bring the most health benefit to all individuals no matter the shape, size, health, diet, or experience level. In other words, PRISE is a comprehensive, holistic and integrative lifestyle of nutrition, fitness and mind/brain health strategies. How to actually "feed" the body with life-giving nutrients, movement and mindfulness is what keeps me coming back. The success stories I hear daily, the response from audiences, the thrill of changing lives for the better, that is a blessed life!

Looking back, if you would have ever asked me when I was eight—that little boy they wanted to put back twice in school and was held in remedial classes— "Do you think *you* would ever, in a million years, become the person who *discovered*, through scientific research, a nutrition and fitness lifestyle program that can work no matter your age, weight, health, fitness level, or even specific diet you follow?" In my mind at the time (and even into adulthood), I would have told you, "No way could that be *me!*" All those years I would have had lots of vibrato with "proof" to back up my postulations: "I could *never* be a scientist, earn not one, but *two* Masters of Science degrees, a doctorate, a post-doctoral fellowship, and *publish* numerous peer-reviewed scientific papers, because I can't even get through middle school without help!" Those degrees and validation have now provided me the credentials to really share my work, so, I smile at what started as my *remedial* life!

Isn't it mind-boggling when *you* look back at your life, because you just never know what the future has in store? I'm sure you have many stories to tell. This leads me to where and why I am here with you today.

Sometimes when I am up in front of these mega-huge audiences I'm still standing there in awe thinking, *Wow, this is really me, I'm really here, and this is really cool!* I never take those opportunities for granted. I'm grateful every time I'm given the platform to share my content, research, and experiences so I may help, even one person in the audience or class. My mission, clearly, is to help as many people as possible achieve optimal health and peak performance every chance I get.

As other educational achievers or graduate and post-graduate people may realize, in attaining advanced degrees, it is often those things that we were told we couldn't do that push us to, perhaps, overachieve. Quite frankly, whether it's business people, entrepreneurs, athletes, skilled craftspeople, or artists, there are a number of people who are told they would never amount to much and, as a result, beat all the odds to become who they are today. I'm no different.

I can only say that if overachieving or overcompensating—with all the advanced degrees, publications, and continued appearances—is what I have done because of my schooling and research, then I can only feel gratitude for the painful obstacles and failures I experienced early in my *remedial* life. I will share more about that at the end of this book. Yes, it is easier to say this now with hindsight! (Should you feel you need to know me more to understand what not only made me this way but has also kept me humble, compassionate, and truly concerned for the well-being of human kind, feel free to skip to part 4, chapter 19.)

My overall goal with this book, and in the coming years, is to continue to educate people, provide resources, give speeches—to as many as will listen—through live audiences and now through the incredible world of the internet and web, social media, media, print, etc. so that others can learn that there *is* an easier way to maintain and attain optimal health and peak performance. I want people to hear it from a real live scientist. Not an "expert" who happened upon something that worked for them alone, not from a "celebrity" who already has a predefined audience, but from a true scientist who through years of research, statistics, experiments, human study, and relationships truly happened upon such amazing results that I can no longer just keep them to myself!

The bottom line is, we all know of people who struggle with ill health or can't make that leap to exercise or lose weight, and because they have gone about it wrong in the past, perhaps because of bad advice or simply just don't know what to do, they have given up. No more! I have written this book in a purposeful, easy-to-read manner and taken my scientist lab coat off to make sure that the studies are easily understood. The value of the research results and recommendations can be executed immediately in your own life. However, should the scientist in you need to read through the scientific studies and data to find your own validations, all the details of research and studies can be found on my websites (www.paularciero.com, www.proteinpacing.com, and www. priseprotocol.com).

By the end of this book you will have the PRISE Life, and, pardon the pun, won the prize. With that "magic" something I call Protein Pacing, you will finally have the chance to be, as they say, the *best* you can be. All the while you will learn about what is entailed in scientific research with terms such as third-party independent research, original investigations, right of first refusal, full disclosure, peer-reviewed, and other facts that will help you to become a discriminating reader and chooser of the type of lifestyle you determine you would like to live. Not a diet. A true healthy and ever-lasting lifestyle. And, as I have said in lectures and articles as I play on Hamlet's words from his famous soliloquy, you *do* have the right "To be or not to be"... healthy. (See, I did learn something from high school after all.)

Most importantly, I want you to *choose* health. Not just survive, but have true optimal health, true life. *La dolce vida*, as they say in Italian. The sweet life. You already have by your willingness to buy my book or listen to my interviews and speeches, now let me motivate you to succeed. You're not alone. There are resources, support systems, products, apps (yes, even mobile phone nutrition/ fitness applications) to help you achieve your goals—one step at a time. And please, have patience with yourself. You don't reach the peak in one try, so finding enjoyment and mental strength along the way can be just as important. That is why I am here to show you the way, *the pace*, for the ultimate *race*: a healthy and vibrant life.

I'm so excited to share all that I have learned and to hear back from each of you on what you found helpful and learned through this book! Change isn't always easy, but you will be shocked by what I learned and how easy it can be.

Don't forget; I'm here for you, so never hesitate to reach out or check the location of my next speech. Come join me. Come join the Protein Pacing and

PRISE Life revolution. And from the bottom of my heart, thank you for being the impetus that made me want to share and find purpose in what has been a lifetime of work.

Finally, remember, the human body is a complicated but perfectly designed mechanism, and we are still in the early stages of understanding everything about it. Embrace it. Embrace your body and type, even as it is today. Embrace your God-given virtue most of all. Embrace the stages and ages of your life. They go by more quickly than you think. Don't lose them to bad information, ill health, and negative emotions. Heed the information and follow the steps and simply believe, because with those few pieces in order you will achieve more than you ever imagined. Take it from a half-a-centurion; don't miss one moment along the way, even *if* life is making other plans for you. One day it will all make sense. And always, always stay positive and, as you will later read, follow my mantra to "Keep your eyes on the prize!"

2

Building Trust

The first job of a leader—at work or at home—is to inspire trust. It's to bring out the best in people by entrusting them with meaningful stewardships, and to create an environment in which high-trust interaction inspires creativity and possibility.
—*Stephen M. R. Covey,* The Speed of Trust:
The One Thing that Changes Everything

The moment there is suspicion about a person's motives, everything he does becomes tainted.
—Mahatma Gandhi

If I have achieved my goal, my first chapter will have read a little like a motivational speech, and I hope the above quotes that start this chapter caught your eye and have you thinking a little. That is because in this chapter I want to work to build your trust in me. Chances are if you have not heard my name yet, you may be a little leery as to what I have to share. I understand. We're human after all, and a bit of skepticism is a healthy way to approach something new. With so much new material coming out in today's fast-paced world, it is really hard to know who to trust. And without breaking down any suspicions you may have in your mind as to my modus operandi and getting the truth to you, ultimately, it will backfire and be a barrier for *your* success in the lifestyle changes you need to make to achieve optimal health and performance.

As I stated in my premise, nature is truly at the core of health, and if we mimic it, we would all be a healthier species. In the most basic sense, scientific methods are simply here to prove that. This section is for the doubter, and I do understand why there are so many of you out there today. If I can get you to understand why my research is so important and accurate, and "create an environment of high-trust" then you and I can, as the young Covey (son of Stephen R. Covey, author of *The 7 Habits of Highly Effective People*) said, "inspire creativity and possibility." This will allow us to make real change in our personal health and well-being and in the health of those we love. It will guarantee success. I meant what I said, that in this stage in life, my greatest rewards are from seeing you succeed.

I am here to share that there are simpler and scientifically proven methods that I have discovered for you to lose weight, stay healthy, nourish your body with the best foods, exercise reasonable amounts of time, and even achieve peak performance if that is what you desire. I'm telling you there is nothing you *can't* do, no matter what shape you are in now, no matter your weight now, and say goodbye to those 500-calorie-a-day total diets and seven hours of intense exercise to lose a few pounds!

I have found the key, the recipe, and while my goal in writing this book is to keep it as easy-to-read as possible, I am going to share some thoughts to keep in mind as you decide whose "scientific" research you believe. The sole reason is that I need you to understand that following the latest and greatest or quickest and flippest diet—or this or that—is not going to serve as a long-term lifestyle solution. So, although there are absolutely some well-qualified fitness trainers, nutritionists, and alternative health practitioners out there, I feel confident enough about my scientific-based research that even they will benefit and eventually adopt what the medical, science, and media communities have already embraced from my research and what I am going to share in this book.

I want to help you learn that there is a huge difference between a "hunch" a physician or fitness trainer or even celebrity may have come upon that might help a portion of the population and a true scientific discovery that will help nearly *all* of the population, if done properly. It is a problem that a lot of material out there has no scientific backing, and the "experts" are simply self-proclaimed. They are either coming up with a diet, fitness strategy of their own through personal experience or they are borrowing from other sources (scientists, personal trainers, celebs, etc.) with no real science to back up their statements.

I am talking about a lifestyle and fitness approach that can work with practically any diet out there. Why? Because I have the scientific proof that has been meticulously gathered for over thirty-plus years of *independent, third-party peer-reviewed science.* This was not a quick find (although it can be a quick fix for some); therefore, you will never experience a quick exit. It will never fall in the "diet fad" category.

There are few, if any, nutrition-exercise scientists who have written a book that contains this much scientific proof on the combined benefits of nutrition and fitness on optimal health and peak performance, so I am asking you to try to look at health from a new perspective, and I'm giving you the unbelievably great news that it doesn't have to be as hard as we have been led to believe! Now *that's* motivating! I am giving you, as an actual scientist, who discovered and conducted the research and the research passed with flying colors, all the strict checks and balances required of high-quality research, including institutional review board (IRB) approval, human subjects' approval, collaborative institutional training certifications, peer-review publications, etc., and, my work has now become the leading material quoted by other researchers in nutrition and applied physiology. I am the "go-to" scientist and content-expert for leading media sources (TV, radio, magazine, newspaper, and internet). You see, I am providing you the actual roadmap that I developed with my research team. I hope by sharing this I am building your trust.

I want to start to teach you to look behind the scenes of other nutrition and exercise programs and develop a discriminating eye by learning more about the "research" that is behind these new celeb diets, training fads, or quick fixes. I am convinced it will help you put your trust in me. Don't forget you can check out my full list of published research in PubMed[4], Google Scholar[5], and on my website at www.priseprotocol.com[6] to learn more for yourself. But to add to the studies, I have spoken to live audiences all over the world, including over 15,000 people at a time, in Las Vegas recently, with a live stream of an additional 17,000. I have received numerous accolades for my discoveries that now, through personal and peer outreach, have already reached several millions of people with additional access by print, magazine articles, published scientific journal articles, media,

---

4 "Arciero P. - PubMed - NCBI," National Center for Biotechnology Information, accessed March 16, 2018, https://www.ncbi.nlm.nih.gov/pubmed/?term=arciero%2Bp.

5 Google, accessed March 17, 2018, https://scholar.google.com/scholar?start=0&q=arciero pj&hl=en&as_sdt=0,3.

6 My research has reached the coveted status of "classic" for being cited over one hundred times by other scientists in peer-reviewed publications and cited well-over three thousand times by other researchers.

TV, radio, blogs, ezines, company newsletter feature articles, etc. Finally, the live radio, taped podcasts, and taped radio shows for interviews are growing exponentially, and people are starting to get the message while now recognizing the name behind the "curtain." Not to forget, I have attained over a million dollars of research funding…and have discovered, yes, actually discovered, new and exciting proof as to how the human body responds to nutrition and exercise. I published my first peer-reviewed research study on how our body metabolizes food back in 1988! This is why I've been nicknamed everything from the pioneer of Protein Pacing to "Dr. Metabolism". However, when I market my brain child, my evangelism of what is now known as Dr. Paul's PRISE Protocol using Protein Pacing on achieving optimal health and peak performance, along with my PRISE app[7] to go with it, I am thrilled to share everything, because I know it will change your life too.

Overall, my research has already been heard firsthand by live audiences (in person or on TV and radio) by millions upon millions of people. When it is pointed out to me how extensive my message and influence has been over the years, I almost get overwhelmed, but the exciting part is that as being one of only a small number of experts in the health and fitness space having this level of influence and impact on others' optimal health and peak performance, I can look at this as birthing a new revolution in health and fitness, and that makes me feel like that really proud papa.

As I work on the parts of this book and am putting the masses of studies and materials together, it is almost too much to embrace. This is why I have sorted through the most important messages and am sharing them right here in this book. When I think hard enough about it, I truly feel this book and venture is just the beginning of the change we can all make. So, my apologies, if this comes across as hubris, but I am really trying to share the incredible impact my research has had on so many and how badly I want it to change your life too.

One of the most astonishing results of my research still stands: Much of what we are being taught and told to do in the area of nutrition and fitness has missed the target and may actually be causing more harm to our bodies versus healing and strengthening us. Every time I share my results in front of audiences they are astounded and shockingly surprised—in a good way—at what I have

---

7   The PRISE app was formerly known as Geniofit. https://itunes.apple.com/us/app/geniofit/ id1087668497?mt=8

discovered and how easy I make it for them to understand and begin to use in their everyday life. They have been asking me for years to get this into the hands of the public and to have a book that they can "take away" to serve as a roadmap to the process.

It is an honor to share these thirty-plus years focused on nutrition, health, wellness, and fitness lifestyle interventions to understand the effects on a human beings' optimal health and peak performance. This means that I have studied and discovered leading research on performance nutrition (fitness, sports, and athletics) and supplementation for not only optimal health but also optimal physical and mental performance. I have also discovered that the timing and understanding of protein and when to consume it to enhance any "diet" you may be currently following as the key ingredient.

I will discuss the process in much greater detail in parts 2 and 3 if you need to skip forward, but soon you will understand I am all about lifestyle changes and not "diets." I am boldly telling you, with scientific proof to back this up, that my Protein Pacing and PRISE Protocol discovery will unequivocally help you with any diet that you choose, such as low-carb, low-fat, gluten-free, paleo, ketogenic, fat-adapted, USDA My Plate, MIND, Intermittent fasting, Mayo, plant-based, veganism, Atkins, DASH, Mediterranean, Metabolic Code, Plant Paradox, Weight Watchers, Jenny Craig, Volumetrics, Ornish, Flat Belly, Nutrisystem, Slimfast, South Beach, Zone, Acid-Alkaline, Fast, Raw/Macrobiotic, Dukan, Whole30, and on and on. Therefore, it will become an easily integrated lifestyle choice for you once you understand just how it works. I truly believe that like the millions of people I have converted, you will too. You will just "get it," and it will come so easily and make so much sense you will not only implement it but, dare I say, even enjoy it.

The bottom line is that no one is happier than when they feel healthy and look great. It's how we as humans are supposed to be. This, unfortunately, is not even close to how the majority of people feel today, and that is an absolute travesty. We are living in an age of sky-rocketing cancer, diabetes, obesity, heart disease, and the list goes on. While pharmaceutical drugs are on the rise and the number of pills people take have increased to astronomical amounts, we as a population are the sickest ever. "Almost 70 percent of Americans take at least one prescription drug, and more than half take two, according to researchers at the

Mayo Clinic and Olmsted Medical Center."[8] "The most commonly prescribed drugs among those studied were opioids (13 percent), antidepressants (13 percent) and antibiotics (17 percent)"[9]. And even more devastating, according to the Centers for Disease Control and Prevention (CDC), "Drug overdose deaths and opioid-involved deaths continue to increase in the United States. The majority of drug overdose deaths (66%) involve an opioid. In 2016, the number of overdose deaths involving opioids (including prescription opioids and heroin) was 5 times higher than in 1999. From 2000 to 2016, more than 600,000 people died from drug overdoses. On average, 115 Americans die every day from an opioid overdose."[10] There is a huge problem with these facts and the reason why I am, in essence, the creator of new paradigms to living healthy lifestyles. I feel strongly that the addiction to pain medicines is coming from ill health; exhaustion, physically and mentally; lack of nutrition; and depression because in a sedentary life your body can't create the "happy" highs that come with healthy and fun exercise. Good nutrition is the key. This all must change, and soon.

What I'm most excited about is how leading research universities and health-care organizations in the world have embraced and cited my research including, National Institutes of Health, Harvard, Stanford, University of Missouri, Columbia, Duke University Medical Center, University of Copenhagen, Mayo Clinic, University of Michigan, University of Maryland, Florida State University, and Ohio State University. More importantly, the type of research I conduct is often performed by only the most well-equipped and funded large-scale research laboratories and institutions due to the "long-term" intervention study design protocols I utilize with my research. For example, most of my research studies involve following and closely monitoring study participants on an exercise and/or nutrition protocol for as short as a couple of weeks to as long as fifteen months! This requires an enormous time and resource commitment by me as the principal investigator, research colleagues, my entire research team, the funding agency, the participants, and the institution. I'm grateful I've had the support of all of these groups over my thirty-year career.

8   Chris Elkins, "Hooked on Pharmaceuticals: Prescription Drug Abuse in America," DrugWatch, July 29, 2015, accessed January 8, 2018, https://www.drugwatch.com/2015/07/29/drug-abuse-in-america/.

9   Ibid.

10   "Opioid Overdose," Centers for Disease Control and Prevention, August 30, 2017, accessed January 8, 2018, https://www.cdc.gov/drugoverdose/epidemic/index.html.

I have learned there is good and bad research out there, so make sure that whatever source you choose to believe that there are "no-strings attached" for the scientist to produce favorable results. Make sure it is independent and autonomous from the funding agency during the entire study process and that relationships are fully disclosed when appropriate. Make it a point to delve a little deeper and spot research that is non-biased, scientifically rigorous, and completely ethical.

Remember, the type of science behind certain nutrition and fitness products is also important depending on whether it's primary versus secondary research. For example, certain companies only rely on research that "other" scientists have conducted and then make claims about their products based on this other research. As consumers, we should be sleuths regarding how and where the claims of certain products are made. If the work is never brought to a level of peer-review then how accurate or truthful is it really? Therefore, the process of peer review, with other scientists from around the world at the top of their game and the most respected in their field, is to carefully pour through the data to determine if it is valid and worthy of publication.

I want you to learn to be a bit of a critical thinker yourself, because in the end this is your body or the body of your loved one. You need to know the research behind the nutrition and exercise program you are choosing. I know we all need some skepticism in our hearts; it keeps us from jumping on the bandwagon that might be taking you down the wrong path because of excellent advertising. But in the essence of my being, I want to prove my scientific and ethical worthiness up front to create relationships built from a foundation of truth and honesty. Nothing speaks stronger than validated scientific research, and the longer it has been around the more authority it inherently gains. If I can build your trust now, you will pay more attention to the details I present in part 3, and it will be easier for you to commit to the entire program—one that works perfectly in sync. I don't want you to throw in the hit or miss pieces someone might have told you to do because they think a section works better their way. I want you to experience the joy of how perfectly this lifestyle works in its totality and to then follow it!

I appreciate you hanging in with me with my lab coat on and letting me at least share a little about scientific research. You will now even be able to throw out some key phrases like *independent, third-party peer-reviewed science.* This is crucial when determining what type of program you are going to implement in your new lifestyle, but most importantly, we are now a trusting and more knowledgeable team—actually a dream team! My vision is for us to create an environment using this roadmap, the PRISE Life Protocol, to achieve optimal health and peak performance. I want to encourage these high-trust interactions to inspire creativity and possibility. It's what I have always aspired to, and I'm not stopping now. In the end, trust and doing your best for others is what nourishes the soul, and that is what I constantly work to achieve. After all, even Ronald Reagan said, "Trust, but verify," and in this case, I whole-heartedly agree.

3

The "Fast-Food" Paradox

A human body is a conversation going on, both within the cells and between the cells, and they're telling each other to grow and to die; when you're sick, something's gone wrong with that conversation.
—W. Daniel Hillis

Nourishing the body and nourishing the soul are the constants we as human beings need to work on throughout our lifetimes. It is a daily process, and we need to remain vigilant because if we let too much time go by without doing both, our quality of life suffers. This is why I am passionate about nurturance, with all its different facets, and committed to making sure the truth behind the science is revealed to you.

By presenting these facts, I want to help you learn to listen to your body, to "mind" your body, and encourage you to follow the steps I've created to help you function and perform the best for the level you are at in this moment. Then, I will help you with your goal to become healthier and stronger and to achieve optimal health. As a result, you will probably exceed the performance level you initially dreamed of. Forearmed with some basic working knowledge as to the importance of learning information from an actual scientist who has spent years researching in a lab, and is teaching you to establish a distinguishing eye, it is now important to help you sort through the masses of information on metabolism, various diets, and why there is so much inaccurate—"fake" news—on how nutrition works and, most importantly, what it means to actually *nourish* ourselves. Hint: It is not with the plastic-covered chemical concoctions, microwaved and fast foods, or other processed things that we consume while washing them down with the diet soft drinks and other "energy drinks."

Look around. A lot of people today are not happy with their weight and are classified as obese—an alarming epidemic growing internationally—not only because of what people consume or because of their lack of exercise but also because of the lack of actual nutrients ingested for their systems to function and live off of. With all the contamination in the air we breathe, the contaminated water we drink, the nutrient-robbed soil from which we harvest our food, to the overindulgences, our bodies can't even get rid of trapped toxins that are stored in our body fat, (especially our belly fat), so how are we supposed to retain and make use of nourished cells. We are filling our "hunger" with nutritionless products, and our bodies just can't figure out how to work properly, forget efficiently. It has become such an epidemic that the term *malobesity* has been coined. It refers to the individual who is malnourished due to heavy empty calories but has excess body fat (obesity). This epidemic didn't even exist twenty years ago; now look at us.

When I look at the population today it tugs at my heart strings because there is no need for this much illness in the world. Our bodies' internal signals have gotten confused and are shooting out quick responses in fear and flight because they don't know what else to do. By consuming these large amounts of highly processed, high-calorie and packaged foods, we are completely deficient in the nutrients, vitamins, and minerals needed for our poor bodies to operate properly. We are silently killing ourselves. The body that is supposed to oversee glucose maintenance and signal insulin to do its job but is so bombarded with toxins, develops diabetes. I'm all too familiar with this. Back in 1993 I conducted a short-term 10 day study with a group of obese men and women with mild type 2 diabetes and showed that small changes in either protein intake or physical activity can drastically improve their glucose and insulin levels and, thus, overall health."[11] This study was groundbreaking and made national news because it demonstrated the power of even short-term lifestyle changes on our overall health. According to the American Diabetes Association, "In 2015, 30.3 million Americans, or 9.4% of the population, had diabetes,"[12] and "1.5 million Americans are diagnosed with diabetes every year."[13] A chart from the Centers

11 PJ Arciero, MD Vukovich, JO Holloszy, SB Racette and WM Kohrt. Comparison of short-term diet and exercise on insulin action in individuals with abnormal glucose tolerance. J Appl Physiol 86:1930-1935, 1999.

12 "Statistics About Diabetes," American Diabetes Association, accessed February 23, 2018, http://www.diabetes.org/diabetes-basics/statistics/.

13 "CDC Newsroom." Centers for Disease Control and Prevention. July 18, 2017. Accessed February 23, 2018. https://www.cdc.gov/media/releases/2017/p0718-diabetes-report.html.

for Disease Control and Prevention (CDC) shows that around 1996 there were about 8 million diabetics and by 2015 about 23 million.[14] The incidences have nearly tripled in under twenty years! Most troubling is that this statistic doesn't even include those who have diabetes but don't know; they are undiagnosed. This statistic alone should make you cringe. Then, take a look at our cholesterol and cardiovascular markers, which are through the roof, keeping heart disease the number one cause of death.[15] These facts alone are more than little clues; these are shocking revelations that can't be ignored. Doesn't this prove that with all these "new and improved" exercise and diet programs out there, somehow we are still missing the mark? We aren't getting healthier; we are getting sicker.

I'm here to say we are most definitely missing the key ingredient to a nutrition and exercise protocol and to point out where and why the errors are happening so you can give your beautiful body a chance to heal and even thrive again. There is *no* life when your days are wracked with pain and illness, or you have difficulty breathing or moving. When you've tried every diet and exercise program out there and still just can't seem to get any better, or even lose a few pounds, no wonder you feel defeated. I feel defeated for you.

You are not even totally to blame.

I'm here to tell you that I don't want you to have to suffer another day. My "heart" can't take it! I want you to follow the steps, believe in me, believe in my scientific proof, and start to understand what metabolism and the body is really all about so you can make permanent changes and enjoy all the fantastic things a healthy body has to offer.

Understand, it is the lack of nourishment, along with lack of exercise (both quality and quantity), that is why we are losing the battle to illness. With the misinformation readily available, we are quickly getting sicker. That is scary. We live in what we think is an educated world, and we have access to quick information that can easily be disseminated, but instead our quality time is being lost due to lack of energy, overeating or self-medicating, all because our bodies are craving nutrients or *life power*, or as ACSM says, *energy balance*, to work. While we spend way too much time on our computers, phones, or sitting

---

14 "US Data & Trends Redirect," Centers for Disease Control and Prevention, April 04, 2012, accessed February 23, 2018, https://www.cdc.gov/diabetes/statistics/slides/long_term_trends.pdf.

15 "National Center for Health Statistics," Centers for Disease Control and Prevention, March 17, 2017, accessed February 23, 2018, https://www.cdc.gov/nchs/fastats/leading-causes-of-death.htm.

watching TV versus getting up and moving, all these actions combine to form a deadly, or at minimum toxic, environment.

America, a "civilized" nation that spends billions on pharmaceuticals, now has a pressing issue with alcohol and drug abuse, from heroine, marijuana, to oxycodone, and is falling rapidly down into the lower percentile—nineteenth according to the WHO of health and medical care. As a matter of fact, "The U.S. health system spends a higher portion of its gross domestic product than any other country but ranks 37 out of 191 countries according to its performance,"[16] which is beyond sad. Longevity is actually decreasing, and health is not getting any better. Somehow, we are making the same poor decisions every day.

"How could that be?" you may ask, because you follow the government recommended heart healthy diet? You might think, *Who am I supposed to believe? Do I trust the low-fat, heart-healthy diets; the low-carb, high-protein, and fat diets that encourage red meat, butter, bacon, and full cream; the high-fiber, high-carb diets; or the no meat, vegetable only diet?* Or do you try the gluten-free, paleo, ketogenic, fat-adapted, low-carb, low-fat, USDA My Plate, MIND, Mayo, plantbased, veganism, Atkins, DASH, Mediterranean, Weight Watchers, Plant Paradox, Jenny Craig, Metabolic Code, Volumetrics, Ornish, Flat Belly, Nutrisystem, Slimfast, South Beach, Zone, Acid-Alkaline, Fast, Raw/Macrobiotic, Dukan, Whole30 diet, and on and on. You get it. There are so many to choose from; it's no wonder most people are utterly confused.

That's why I am here to help you learn. I am going to teach you a lifestyle that supersedes but can work with all diets out there. But just as important even teach you in part 2 what types of foods should become your go-tos and what type and how much exercise is ideal. Let me start first though with just a little primer to keep in your head as you go along and one that is important to share with your friends. I call it the "Slow and Dirty Rules for Optimal Health," because just following this with a few other food tricks (keys) from this chapter will get you primed for what has now been popularly called, Dr. Paul's PRISE Protocol.

Recently, people have been talking about "slow" vs. "fast" food, and my brother-in-law reminded me with a question he had that not everyone is familiar with this concept. I've been a proponent of the "slow food" philosophy for years, but more people are familiar with the term "fast food." Essentially, "fast

---

16   "World Health Organization Assesses the World's Health Systems," WHO, accessed January 8, 2018, http://www.who.int/whr/2000/media_centre/press_release/en/.

food" is exactly what the name implies—food that's been (mass) produced faster than its "natural life cycle through the use of artificial stimulants, such as fertilizers, over/forced-feeding methods, pesticides, hormones, growth factors, and genetically modified organisms.

Fast food is the main staple in "fast-food" restaurants and convenience stores, but it's also abundant in traditional grocery stores. Fast food may also come in the form of conventional produce (fruits, vegetables, grains), animal products (milk, eggs, meat, etc.), and just about every prepackaged, processed food. Whatever the shape, size, and type of fast food, it's usually been mass-produced in tightly confined living quarters, such as a cage or feed lot, or in high-yield single-crop farms. Ironically, the shortened and stimulated production "life cycle" of fast food results in a strangely prolonged shelf life, once the food is harvested and brought to market. In other words, fast food is produced quickly but lives long. (Think of the Twinkie with the urban legend twenty-plus-year shelf life!)

Herein lies the hidden danger of fast food. The longer-than-normal shelf life wreaks havoc on the human body, because the harmful chemicals used to protect and stimulate the growth of the vegetable, fruit, grain, or animal gets passed on to the cells in our body. Many experts believe these synthetic chemicals contribute to the current plague of modern-day diseases, such as cardiovascular and metabolic disease, certain cancers, as well as inflammatory and neurodegenerative disorders.

I call it the "fast-food paradox"—a shortened life cycle and a prolonged shelf life (after life). Slow food, on the other hand, is the exact opposite. It includes foods that have been grown and raised without the use of harmful toxins and artificial growth factors and protectants, and thus require a longer life cycle to grow and mature. Once they have undergone their natural course of growth, their shelf life is usually very short.

Examples of slow food include local and/or organic produce, free-range, grass-fed beef, dairy, eggs, and poultry, as well as most wild seafood. You're probably thinking, *If it's local, it must be "fast?"* Actually, local produce (vegetables and fruits) and animal-based products mature according to the timeline that nature intended. Therefore, it comes to market and, eventually your dinner table, long after conventional food sources arrive.

Slow food is characterized by an extended, natural life cycle and a brief shelf life (after life), so you need to restock more often. This is a good thing. As such, there is limited, if any, exposure to harmful toxic residues entering our cells. Slow food is rich in nutrients and other healthy chemicals called antioxidants and polyphenolic compounds, all of which protect our bodies from disease.

Local farmers markets, community-supported agriculture (CSA), home gardens/farms, and clean oceans and fresh water streams/lakes are ideal sources for much of your staple food items. These are also where you will find the healthiest sources of "dirty" whole foods. "Dirty" means, most of the food we eat should come directly from the earth and sea—think vegetables, grains, beans, fruits, seeds/nuts, and animal foods (fish, meat, eggs, dairy).

Much less of the food we eat should come from a "clean" wrapped package, unless it is a high quality nutrient-dense engineered food. These can be some of the healthiest foods we can eat. Highly processed fast food often appears sterile, refined, and shiny, and is referred to as "clean" food. Some health professionals confuse "eating clean" with eating healthy. However, "clean" applies much better to the fast-food production process and should be minimized. The point is, at any moment during the day, you have a choice between nutrient-dense slow and dirty food, including nutrient-dense engineered food, or fast food. I want you to do everything in your power to choose nutrient-dense slow and dirty food (including engineered) and eat it often. Having said all of that, I'm also one of the first scientists to include a "cheat day" in my research studies with phenomenal results! I did this because I will be the first person to say, perfection is impossible, and allowing ourselves the occasional treat when it comes to food is one way to keep us on track. In my PRISE Life Cookbook (coming out soon), I detail my 85%–15% Rule. This simply means 85% of the time try to eat healthy, dirty foods, and the other 15% indulge in your favorite comfort foods. To make this even easier to follow using my Protein Pacing plan, simply include one "cheat meal" a day, or set aside one day each week to indulge. Either way, this adheres to my 85%–15% Rule. But remember, stay within the same number of total calories for each "cheat meal or day" that you would normally follow eating healthy.

While we are on the topic of eating fresh slow food and eating dirty, I want you to also think of applying this to other parts of your life that expose your body to toxins. It could be the crazy "clean" concoctions in shampoo or skin cream. It could be "fresh and clean"-scented air fresheners, cleaning products, toothpaste, you name it. But they are all filled with chemicals that may harm, not heal, your body. They are just as dangerous to your cells as the foods we ingest.

The wonderful news is that I have come upon a way that even if we have exposed ourselves, intentionally or unintentionally, to these toxins there is a way to eat properly to increase the rate at which you expel toxins. It is an incredible process I discovered and called Protein Pacing along with another popular concept, intermittent fasting. There is so much more I want to teach you about it, but I just want you to *hear*, or rather familiarize, yourself with the term for now so when you get to the material in parts 2 and 3, you will already be prepped and pumped to comply with my advice. This process and protocol is crucial to your optimal health, so I'm going to share a little "teaser" next.

I am pretty much the first to discuss the relationship between weight loss, toxins, and oxidative stress through scientific measures. [17,18,19,20] It is exciting to realize that we now have scientific evidence that the quality of your diet does matter! Through diet, we can favorably support the detoxification process, oxidative stress levels, and blood vessel health, all while enhancing weight loss. This major study of mine in particular was cited by Science Daily on January 11, 2017 which stated, "Research by exercise scientists has found that a balanced, protein-pacing, low-calorie diet that includes intermittent fasting not only achieves long-term weight loss, but also helps release toxins in the form of polychlorinated biphenyls (PCBs) from the body fat stores, in addition to enhancing heart health and reducing oxidative stress." [21] In case you don't know what and how detrimental they are, PCBs are a group of organic compounds

17 Feng He, Li Zuo, Emery Ward, and Paul Arciero (Senior Corresponding Author). "Serum Polychlorinated Biphenyls Increase and Oxidative Stress Decreases with a Protein-Pacing Caloric Restriction Diet in Obese Men and Women." *International Journal of Environmental Research and Public Health* 14, no. 12 (2017): 59. doi:10.3390/ijerph14010059.

18 Paul Arciero et al., "Protein-Pacing Caloric-Restriction Enhances Body Composition Similarly in Obese Men and Women during Weight Loss and Sustains Efficacy during Long-Term Weight Maintenance," *Nutrients* 8, no. 12 (2016): doi:10.3390/nu8080476.

19 Li Zuo, Feng He, Grant M. Tinsley, Benjamin K. Pannell, Emery Ward, and Paul J. Arciero. "Comparison of High-Protein, Intermittent Fasting Low-Calorie Diet and Heart Healthy Diet for Vascular Health of the Obese." *Frontiers in Physiology* 7 (2016). doi:10.3389/fphys.2016.00350.

20 Skidmore College. "Diet helps shed pounds, release toxins and reduce oxidative stress." ScienceDaily. ScienceDaily, 11 January 2017. Available at: www.sciencedaily.com/releases/2017/01/170111184102.htm.

21 "OECD Statistics." OECD Statistics. Accessed March 7, 2018. https://stats.oecd.org/glossary/detail.asp?ID=2078.

used in the manufacture of plastics, as lubricants, and dielectric fluids in transformers, in protective coating for wood, metal, and concrete, and in adhesives, wire coating and so forth. They are highly toxic to aquatic life and persist in the environment for long periods of time. They can accumulate in food chains and may produce harmful side effects at high concentrations."[22] The extent to which our world has become contaminated by these is mind-boggling.

We know we need to reduce exposure to these toxins, but how proactive are we about this? Have we become complacent because we are too tired to care? Or have we just become "frozen," unable to move because we truly have no clue as to the direction that is best for our bodies, especially with all the latest and greatest diets coming out? Well, I am here to share some amazing news and to *un*-paralyze you!

With the smallest of efforts by humans to improve their own miraculous creation, by eating a certain way, what we found was that the body actually *compensated*, took over, worked on its own by *increasing* disease-fighting antioxidants and *decreasing* cellular-damaging oxidative stress. This is astounding. In response to this flood of PCBs, the body was coming to its own defense, likely scavenging and squelching the toxins. It is because of this we had a healthy weight-loss intervention for all the participants in the research study. That's an important public health message, and it is being missed in a lot of the fad diets used out there. It is yet another reason why my PRISE Protocol that includes Protein Pacing and intermittent fasting will last long after others have been forgotten—but you will want to follow it precisely. No reinventing the wheel needed. It is designed to help your body release toxins from your stored body fat, which in turn will help you lose weight and feel great.

I also want to take a minute to discuss "whole foods" because I am clarifying some terms like dirty vs. clean foods, and I want to make sure we are completely in sync. When I talked about growing your own food source from the earth's soil ultimately being the greatest source of nourishment to keep our bodies healthy and functioning at the highest level, I meant it. Mother Earth is, undoubtedly, still the prime nourisher, and if we focus on the quality of unadulterated soil and nutrients found within, as originally created, we as a species will thrive again. The problem is the soils are so depleted and we are eating so much genetically

---

22   Ibid.

modified and manufactured food that we have got to replace the nutrients that have been taken away from us. We have to focus on high-quality (whole) foods, in order to become a healthier world.

The pressing question, and one I know you are probably wondering about is, "What about these new *packaged* nutritional diets? Are they even good for you?" To keep you motivated, and on board, I want to comment. I believe we can obtain optimal nourishment from both high-quality whole foods as well as powders, bars, and meal replacements that must contain naturally sourced high-quality ingredients. I refer to this as "nutrient-dense engineered" food as opposed to "nutrient-deficient engineered" food that are loaded with artificial sweeteners or refined sugar, sodium and lacking in fiber and nutrients. Some would say all meat, vegetables, fruits, dairy, etc. are whole foods so they must be good for us; however, the manner in which they are grown (heavy pesticides, insecticides, etc.), cultivated (genetically modified organism [GMO] etc.), and cared for (caged, grain-fed, etc.) make a huge difference and sometimes are less healthy than high-quality "packaged goods," meal replacements, and supplements or "nutrient-dense engineered" foods. I'm essentially saying that I know the quality of a certain *few* nutritional supplement companies that source the *best* ingredients in their bars, powders, meal replacements, vitamins/minerals, etc. that are of higher quality than many "whole foods." After years of research and personal interest, I have found the ones that truly can step up your health with *the proper* and needed *combinations* of complementary vitamins, minerals, and phytonutrients (plant nutrients). They are not packed with sugar, and they don't just throw in a smidgen of an ingredient to be able to make fancy claims like this product contains methylsulfonylmethane (MSM)[23] and ginseng; therefore, it is a "nutritional" drink or bar.

Now that I've thrown at you trying to eat slow and dirty food, whole foods and the fact that I am not against nutritional supplementation and meal replacements, and in case I've overwhelmed you, here is the great news: To achieve optimal health, you need your cells to be nurtured, and *any* change you make on a daily basis with this philosophy is going to pay off. One less diet soda, one

---

23   An herb touted to help with arthritis and joint pain but has many different uses. It has been studied by the National Institutes of Health (NIH) for osteoarthritis. "Dimethyl Sulfoxide (DMSO) and Methylsulfonylmethane (MSM) for Osteoarthritis." National Center for Complementary and Integrative Health. September 24, 2017. Accessed February 23, 2018. https://nccih.nih.gov/health/supplements/dmso-msm.

less fast food, one less high-calorie, sodium-rich, prepackaged meal, one well-documented and researched healthier supplementation product, one less sugar and caffeine-packed energy drink, one less spray of "fresh air" or chemical perfume, and you are well on your way to creating healthier habits that will pay off in the near future.

A wonderful side effect of this new type of eating is that soon you are going to find the taste of fake food and smell of fake scents "off," and you will start craving more flavorful, earth-based, healthful food and natural essences. How fun that finally "dirty" is a good word. These small steps alone are going to help your metabolism and body's healing in ways you would never believe, so please trust me on this as you wrap your head around and rev up to start the program that I created for "life."

With the whole food, slow and dirty food engrained in your subconscious nudging you to do what is right, we will next move on to Human Metabolism 101. But always remember that at the core, do say yes to dirty whole foods, nutrient-dense engineered food and no to clean, refined, prepackaged, "nutrient-deficient" chemical foods. Your body will help you release toxins quicker than you might have ever believed. Let's really commit to *nourishing* our bodies and finally let the cells have a healthy communication chain. With clear, natural, and healing channels, a dramatic change and increased vitality are bound to bless you. I promise you, by implementing these small steps, even the weakest bodies can start to declog, detox, and get healthy.

4

Walk This Whey:
Busting Diet Myths

The point of modern propaganda isn't only to misinform or push an agenda. It is to exhaust your critical thinking, to annihilate truth.
Garry Kasparov—13th World Chess Champion

I don't think you can go a few days in the media without hearing someone's opinion on fasting, juicing, cleansing, supplementation, etc., so I'm going to share some of my findings and beliefs up front, because I have *scientific proof for the answers*. I am not just guessing because it is the trend or the hot topic. Some, inappropriately, call it myth-busting because often some of these "facts" have some truth to them, which is why they can build up so much hype in the media. With that said, I want to first address issues related to intermittent fasting.

Metabolism is primarily defined as the sum total of all chemical reactions occurring in all of the cells to help us maintain bodily functions at rest. A significant portion of our metabolism is focused on trying to protect our cells from harmful invaders, such as toxins. One very popular lifestyle strategy that has gained enormous attention is intermittent fasting, sometimes referred to as nutritional cleansing. Specifically, intermittent fasting is often associated with helping the body to restore, replenish, and heal and recently has even showed signs of slowing down aging in humans! The reason is our bodies naturally go through cycles of breaking down and building up as well as periodic "house cleaning." The ideal scenario/environment for the body to perform its "house cleaning" is a similar process we use in our own homes. The best time to house clean is when there is not a lot of clutter, basically an empty house. Inside of our bodies, intermittent fasting is associated with the best environment to "clean house" and restore optimal function. Intermittent fasting can be accomplished in several different ways:

◊ 16/8 Method: consists of fasting for sixteen hours (no food or caloric drinks, only water) and then eating two or more meals within an eight hour window. Also called time-restricted eating.

◊ 5:2 Method: involves five days of normal eating and two days of fasting that limits calorie intake to 300–600 calories. The two-day fasts can be any two days during the week.

◊ 24-Hour Fast Method: this is the typical fast most people are familiar with, which involves refraining from eating and drinking (water only) with up to 500 calories for a twenty-four-hour period one to two days per week.

◊ Alternate Day Fasting Method: as the name implies, this requires fasting every other day either with no food (water only) or eating up to 500 calories during the fast days.

There are other modifications of these four main types of fasting, such as the fasting mimicking diet, that are the most well-known and followed. While they each provide a slightly different form of intermittent fasting, the 5:2 and 24-Hour Fast methods seem to provide the best environment to achieve the best results if done properly. I recommend the following: if your goal is weight loss, incorporate the 5:2 or 24-Hour Fast methods on a weekly basis up to three months, and then once you've achieved your weight loss goal, aim to fast only one to two days per month. If you're not interested in weight loss, reap the benefits of either of these methods by limiting to one to two days per month. This is the exact intermittent fasting routines I've used in my own research with fantastic results![24] Lastly, and perhaps most importantly, the quality of the 300–600 calories you choose to consume on these intermittent fasting days will "make" or "break" the benefit it provides your body. In other words, paying close attention to ingesting high-quality, nutrient dense, phytochemical (antioxidant/adaptogen)-rich foods is the key to getting the

---

24   Arciero 2016; He et al.; Zuo et al. can be reviewed in full at www.priseprotocol.com.

best results. I have the published research to support this![25]Some of the best sources of antioxidants (substances that prevent damaging oxidative stress reactions in the body) and adaptogens (plant substances that help our bodies adapt to stress) I've used in my research to support intermittent fasting, include blueberries, raspberries, bilberries, turmeric, rhodiola, ashwagandha, bacopa, schizandra, eleuthero, and pau d'arco. Here is a simple and very effective 1-2 day/week intermittent fast (or cleanse) I've used with clients, athletes and study participants: Before Breakfast - multivitamin with adaptogen beverage (25 calories); Breakfast – antioxidant beverage with protein snack (70 calories); Mid-morning Snack – small handful of nuts/seeds and dried fruit (50 calories for women, 100 calories for men); Lunch – antioxidant beverage with protein snack (70 calories); Mid-afternoon Snack – antioxidant beverage with protein snack (70 calories for women, 120 calories for men); Dinner – antioxidant beverage with protein snack and multivitamin (70 calories). This intermittent fast cleanse provides approximately 355 calories for women and 455 calories for men per day.

Some people like to use the term "cleansing" to identify this intermittent fasting period of very low-calorie intake (fasting) to allow the body to fully and properly remove harmful unwanted substances (toxins) that have accumulated. I know it's a funny analogy, but like I said, the same way it is easiest and most effective to clean an empty house, it's also most effective to clean out and restore our bodies to optimal health when there is less food and "junk" in it. At least now you are familiar with my terminology and recommendations.

You will learn in part 3 that in my program I am not asking people to deprive themselves for long periods of time, and I am certainly not asking a diabetic with a blood sugar issue not to eat. I am talking about nourishing the body to a point that when the healthy foods and possible supplements are added they are not just flushed out of the body because they went with all the other goop that has been built up in the bowels or even our organs and tissues.

When we think of cleaning house, people also often mix the words *juicing* with *cleansing*, so I want to take a moment to give you my thoughts on this. All

---

25   Feng He, Li Zuo, Emery Ward, and Paul Arciero (Senior Corresponding Author). "Serum Polychlorinated Biphenyls Increase and Oxidative Stress Decreases with a Protein-Pacing Caloric Restriction Diet in Obese Men and Women." *International Journal of Environmental Research and Public Health* 14, no. 12 (2017): 59. doi:10.3390/ijerph14010059.

the rave these days in nutrition and health is "juicing." But what is juicing, and is it really better for us than the "real deal" of fresh fruits and vegetables? I've already discussed dirty and whole foods, so here goes juicing. Essentially, juicing is the process of extracting out only the juice-containing portion of any fruit or vegetable leaving behind the outer (skin) layer, seeds, and most of the pulp and natural fiber. This results in a liquid-rich cornucopia of health-promoting vitamins, minerals, and other potent bioactive compounds, also known as phyto- (plant-based) chemicals. The most well-known of which are called antioxidants. Antioxidants are often associated with powerful health benefits, such as increased immunity and disease protection, as well as enhanced energy.

There are two main juice-extraction methods: 1) heat-generated and 2) cold-pressed. Much has been written highlighting the differences between the two techniques (heat-generated versus cold-pressed juicers). The heat-generating juicers use a super-fast spinning blade (called centrifugal extractors) against a mesh filter that separates the pulp from the juice. Although not exactly the same thing, as a young boy I remember using a "spinning juicer" with freshly squeezed oranges and grapefruits during the cold winter months—the juice was delicious and always seemed to keep our house of nine people living in close quarters a bit healthier than our friends and neighbors! The limitation of the modern-day juicer is they produce a lot of heat while spinning, which likely destroys the natural enzymes within the fruit and vegetables as well as oxidizes some of the health-promoting nutrients.

Cold-pressed, on the other hand, is considered much gentler because it simply crushes and then presses the fruit and vegetables, retaining nearly all of the enzymes and other health-boosting phyto-chemicals (antioxidants). As a result, the take-away message from many juicing pundits is that cold-pressed is a healthier choice, and I agree. Regardless of the juice-extracting technique used (heat-generated or cold-pressed) they are both susceptible to spoilage due to microorganism growth, thus limiting their shelf life to only two to five days, at most. So, you better drink up fast!

Fortunately, heat pasteurization methods are often used to neutralize the harmful microorganisms that lead to spoilage, which extends the juice life up to forty-five days. However, there is a down side to pasteurization. Similar to heat-generated juice extraction, heat-pasteurization destroys many of the health-promoting properties of the fruit or vegetable juice.

Recently, a new processing technique has been introduced to the "juicing" market that neutralizes harmful microorganisms, and similarly extends juice life (up to forty-five days), but without the negative consequences of typical heat-generated pasteurization. This process is referred to as high-pressure processing or HPP. According to recent food science research, HPP retains many of the original nutrients, flavor, and texture of fruits and vegetables (HPP versus thermal pasteurization). This is reason enough to always choose fresh juices that have been prepared using both cold-pressed and HPP techniques versus standard heat processing and pasteurization.

This brings me to my final point regarding whether to juice or not. Most food science experts would agree that eating the whole fruit or vegetable, especially a local and/or organic version, should be your top priority for optimal health. But, let's face it, our hectic on-the-go lifestyles place convenience at a premium. As such, the quick, convenient, and long shelf life of cold-pressed, HPP juices provide a nourishing alternative to the real deal. Better yet, if you want to enjoy the highest level of nourishment on-the-go, opt for a whole fruit and vegetable-blended smoothie with some added protein. This will provide all of the vitamins, minerals, antioxidants, fiber, and other nutrients contained within the whole fruit and vegetable and will save you money too. Although the whole fruit and vegetable protein smoothie may provide a bit more calories, the fiber and roughage will benefit you more in the end. But remember, if I can encourage you at all in those weak or on-the-run moments, choose "the whole fruit and nothing but the fruit!"

With our house cleaned and juicing addressed, I can't skip over the most important part of my program, which has to do with protein. Everyone is talking these days about protein this, carb that, or fat this, and I will give you all the details, but I want to alert you to the fact that there are more healthy types of protein out there than you may have been led to believe. Because some of them are newer, and again, trending, or hot topics, I would be remiss not to include my thoughts.

Normally when we think of protein we are led to think only animal products, but you will learn that plants sources, including vegetables, grains, nuts, and legumes have protein too. Even some of the "newer" sources that have been created, that people call protein powders, provide excellent sources of protein. Since the invention of these powders and the actual understanding that plants have protein, I am actually not against using them, and even prefer them in some circumstances. However, and this is a big beware note: quality is everything. If they come from good sources of animal foods like whey or collagen, or from plant sources like pea, brown rice, fava, mung, pumpkin seed, tapioca, legumes, or hemp (and some forms of soy) protein, they can help support an excellent diet. But, if they are full of simple and/or fake sugars, mismatched nutrients thrown in, too small to have any healthy benefit, and topped with artificial flavorings and preservatives, run for your life! It's no better than gulping down a fast-food burger and think that you are nourishing yourself! Chances are you will also be hungry in about fifteen minutes after you just finished that "meal."

I always ask myself, "Protein powder, but at what cost?"

The first and perhaps most popular source these days is something called "whey" protein.

But what is *whey*? Ever remember Mother Goose? "Little Miss Muffet, sat on a tuffet, eating her curds and whey." Do you know what this is? It is the lumps and liquid of nothing other than cottage cheese! Yup! And guess what the clumping parts are? Protein curds. And the liquid part? Whey! Now don't say Mother Goose wasn't trying to teach us something! But all joking aside, whey proteins are the by-product—the waste product—that occurs in the production of cheese, but, of course, first you must start with milk. "Milk is made of two proteins, casein and whey. Whey protein can be separated from the casein in milk or formed as a by-product of cheese making."[26] It is important to note that, "Whey protein is considered a complete protein as it contains all 9 essential amino acids (and 11 non-essential amino acids). It is low in lactose content."[27] I talk more about this in the next part when I discuss macronutrients, but for now let's focus on lactose, the sugar component of dairy. A lot of people have issues with dairy, or rather the lactose in dairy, and therefore as these powders have evolved, so has the level of lactose in them. That's why you might have heard terms like concentrate vs. isolate vs. hydrolysate. All this has been created because now you can remove lactose from whey through a process called

---

26 "Medical News Today." Medical News Today. Accessed February 11, 2018. https://www.medicalnews-today.com/articles/263371.php.

27 Ibid.

filtration. This process makes even the lactose intolerant, tolerant.

Filtration is a widespread method and when handled correctly can result in all, but 15% of the lactose being successfully extracted from the whey. The ion exchange process is less affordable and may result in a final product which has all but 5% of the lactose removed. If you really want to get into the nitty-gritty of the process, I recommend *The Dairy Processing Handbook*[28], the chapter on "Whey Processing." But I'm going to share the major points in lay people's terms so let's start with the "concentrate."

Whey protein concentrate is slightly less filtered, the first step, and therefore the least processed than whey protein isolates or hydrolysate. It is usually about 80% protein (watch the brand though because some are as low as 35% and use unhealthy fillers.) Remember, higher is better because it is higher protein by weight. But beware, if you are lactose intolerant, this may still give you problems because there is inherently a larger concentration of lactose in a concentrate. The upside is you are going to have the best immune-boosting support from this least-processed form, and it digests more slowly so it keeps you satiated longer and contains health-boosting micro/macroglobulin proteins and peptides.

If we treat the concentrate more it becomes the second stage and 90% pure protein by weight, often even 95%. Isolate protein supplements undergo several purification processes that filter out virtually all the fat and carbohydrates and due to this are about 95% pure protein by weight. The benefits of whey protein isolate is that it is easily digestible, contains very low amounts of lactose, and also increases protein synthesis allowing for a large spike in amino acid levels. The healthy micro/macroglobulin proteins and peptides in concentrate are not present in isolate, and therefore whey protein concentrate is actually considered healthier, by many experts, than isolate. Almost all the lactose is removed, so good for lactose intolerance, but because it is broken into smaller peptides, you may lose some immune-boosting benefits.

Hydrolyzed protein (hydrolysate), as you have probably seen on labels, are the fastest absorbing because they are already so broken down, but with that you are destroying most of the immune benefits. This was done to remove the allergenic issues for people and also provide the highest amount of protein per volume. Many hard-core body building and fitness models opt for this, but it's

28   "Dairy Processing Handbook." Dairy Processing Handbook. Accessed February 11, 2018. http://dairy-processinghandbook.com/chapter/whey-processing.

not my top choice in terms of overall health benefits.

Some people focus on something called "de"-naturing the protein—you may have heard undenatured and denatured whey protein. Essentially, *undenatured* means the naturally occurring proteins and bioactive compounds have not been altered with chemicals and high-temperature heating during processing. Whereas, *denatured* whey protein has been chemically altered, and, therefore has destroyed these health-promoting compounds in an attempt to produce a more highly concentrated form of whey protein. Based on the available scientific evidence, I highly recommend an undenatured whey protein concentrate. This type of whey protein is in its most natural form and yields many of the health benefits it was intended to provide from nature. Combining undenatured whey protein with a natural-eco-sourced whey protein from grass-fed or pasture-raised cows may add further benefit to the whey by providing a higher concentration and amount of heart and health-boosting omega-3 fatty acids.

In the laboratory, we actually spend time looking and talking about something called the biological value (BV) of protein sources. BV measures how efficiently a protein source is digested and after that utilized in protein synthesis. If all the protein you digest from a certain source is made available to the body to make different proteins, it's incredibly effective and receives a high BV score. The less protein from a certain source that may be made available for protein synthesis receives a lower score.[29]

Fascinating to note that whey protein isolate has a BV score of about 160— the highest BV score of any protein source known to man to date. This is important when you compare this to casein. Raw cow's milk, for example, is 5%–10% protein out of which 80% is casein and 20% whey. What is casein? Casein is the main protein source in milk, accounting for approximately 80% of the protein. Like whey, casein protein has a high BV value that suggests it contains all the essential amino acids required for protein synthesis in your body. Casein is a slow-digesting protein, meaning it takes longer to enter the bloodstream and cells and initiate protein synthesis compared to whey protein, which is very fast acting. The speed of the gastric emptying slows down, meaning acids in casein enter the blood more slowly.

Just one scoop of casein (also called micellar) protein contains a massive 24

29   "National Center for Biotechnology Information." National Center for Biotechnology Information. Accessed February 11, 2018. https://www.ncbi.nlm.nih.gov/pmc/articles/PMC3905294/.

g of protein. Casein allows for the repair and healing of muscle fibers to reduce muscle soreness and increase protein synthesis. Through helping shorten healing time, casein protein can help you increase power and strength and allow you to train harder. By consuming casein, you may get a great source of protein without excess calories, including carbohydrates. Studies show that casein protein may promote weight reduction and decrease excess fat.

It's really important to consider taking casein protein before bed. This type of protein is often recommended as the best nighttime meal. Scientific research shows casein protein may take up to seven hours to digest, which is just about as long as the common person sleeps every single night. Casein extends the release of amino acids to the bloodstream, improving protein (nitrogen) retention and thus the ability to build muscle. Remember, however, that any period spent sleeping is a period when your body is not getting any new nutrients. As you're probably aware, if you run out of amino acids in your bloodstream, your body can start breaking down muscle proteins to fuel itself. Taking casein before going to bed is an effective strategy to avoid protein breakdown and amino acid oxidation. However, there is controversy regarding the health effects of casein protein, and in my opinion, whey is the healthier choice between the two and should be the primary form of your protein intake combined with healthy plant-based sources. I discuss all of this further in part 3.

As for the BV, micellar casein has a BV of 90. Which one is best for muscle development or a lean body composition, you ask? It really depends on your overall goal. If optimal health and peak performance are your top priority, I recommend undenatured whey protein concentrate. If you are solely focused on muscle development, then experiment with casein but always have some source of undenatured whey concentrate in your diet along with the best plant-based proteins.

One more topic before I wrap, is plant-based protein versus animal protein, including whey and casein. Let me start by stating I'm a huge plant-based supporter because of the many proven health and performance benefits of eating a plant-based diet. Having said this, I also want to clearly point out that our bodies respond much better to animal-based protein when it comes to lean muscle mass and fat burning. This is why most of the research supports animal-based protein to maximize body composition. Of all the plant-based proteins, a combination of pea, legume, fava, mung, pumpkin seed, and brown rice protein are the highest quality with other plant-based proteins like hemp and soy showing some health and body composition benefits. Eating pea, legume, fava, mung, pumpkin seed, brown rice, and hemp in powder form are healthy and effective ways to meet your Protein Pacing goals, and I enjoy these myself. Of course, whole food plant-based proteins are excellent sources too, such as legumes like lentils, black beans, chickpeas, and grains like quinoa. However, you'll do best to avoid soy protein powders at all costs, and lean toward collagen protein, because of the processing and higher levels of plant estrogens (phytoestrogens). If you consume soy protein, stay with naturally occurring whole plant sources, such as fermented soy (tofu), edamame, tempeh, miso, and natto.

The bottom line for me, and when I am asked specifically about whey, I respond, "Yes, undenatured whey and concentrate is best," remembering that quality is everything. Whey is a complete protein with amino acids that can turn on protein synthesis and thereby help the muscles and bone/body thrive. Using the right amount at the right time can help you lose weight and gain lean muscle mass, and it's one of my top go-tos for Protein Pacing. It has vital nutrients, and it opens up so many protein options for you to consume that your meals will never get boring and you will stay full longer.

With the masses of information that come across our desks every day, it really is hard to sort through the facts and throw out the fiction. I hope some of my myth-busting and clarifications on intermittent fasting, "house cleaning," biological value of protein, and whey vs. plant proteins such as soy and pea, help you feel more confident about the choices you make every day. In the end, I don't want the truth annihilated or only partial truths told. I am hopeful that my views, with scientific proof to back them up, will help you have the energy to continue to think critically and make the right and informed choices for you and your loved ones. Nothing is worse than watching someone work diligently to be healthy and follow a lifestyle program religiously, only come to find out the basis of the program has absolutely zero facts and is all propaganda.

5

"Mind" Your Body: Serve Up Success

Champions aren't made in the gyms. Champions are made from something they have deep inside them—a desire, a dream, a vision.
—Muhammad Ali, legendary boxer

Having been a successful athlete myself, winning tennis championships to this day, competing in triathlons, road races, a snowshoeing medalist, and playing hockey, I have firsthand experience of what it takes to be a champion. I know that it is a drive and a desire deep within that leads you to dream, as Muhammed Ali so beautifully expressed. Even more than that, as a scientist who studied human physiology, nutrition, and neuropsychology, I know there are mysteries of the mind that go way beyond what numbers and statistics could ever tell us. As analytical as I am, I have a deeper belief in spiritual concepts. I believe in using every power possible to gain the *advantage*.

Games can be won or lost in our minds well before we show up for a competition, and that is what this chapter is all about. This chapter is about you setting your mind right, right this second, so that you will no longer ever need another diet, you will no longer ever lose health, and so that you, starting today, are going to finally win the challenge to reach your peak fitness and physical performance. I have all the tools you need so I am hypnotizing, programing, and encouraging you with these very words—with the backing of the universe. *Today* is the day, with this book in hand, you will throw away the bad material and fad diets and create a maintainable and healthy lifestyle that will help you achieve optimal health and fitness. Repeat that. "*Today* is the day, with this book in hand, I will throw away the bad material and fad diets and create a maintainable and healthy lifestyle that will help me achieve optimal health and fitness." Believe it.

In something called the Abraham-Hicks trainings, which teaches about the laws of attraction and explains that you are your own creator with every *thought*, they drive a nutritional and fitness point home with the following teaching: "Metabolism is a vibrational response to a moment in time. Metabolism is the way energy is moving through your body, you see. And so 'everything' is in response to the way you feel. Everything is. Everything is mind over matter."[30,31] If we accept that we have a deeper influence over what happens to our metabolism, as I believe we also have over what happens to our health, fitness, and wellness, then this is reason all the more we need to be careful what we think and especially what we say. We need to seriously consider who we keep around us, because negative people breed negative energy, and there is no time for your metabolism, your mind, or your body to pick up any of those sensations from limited-thinking or uninformed individuals. In fact, new research out of Harvard University shows happiness is truly contagious, but so are obesity and smoking! So choose your company wisely! When you have mastered this, you will succeed in the lifestyle changes I am teaching you.

When you have conquered the lifestyle changes, you will then be able to teach others and maybe then, even help those naysayers. Until that day, I am asking you to be aware, surround yourself by others who can love you unconditionally, and learn to love yourself as you are in this moment, knowing, soon, very soon, you will be the best you, ever.

The mental side of optimal health and peak performance is just as important as the physical side, because not only does it help you develop deep spiritual commitments that "tune you up" for success but it also helps you become aware of what your body is saying to you. Your mind will entice you by making you find nutrient-dense, high-quality foods more attractive, it will nudge you when you are down and show you the value of mood-enhancing endorphins when you exercise so that you will want more of all the "good" stuff, and it will even tell you when today is a day for rest.

Vince Lombardi said, "Perfection isn't attainable, but if we chase perfection

---

30   "Abraham-Hicks Sessions, accessed February 1, 2018, https://abrahamhickssessions.wordpress. com//2014/07/11/metabolism-is-vibrational-response-2/.

31   To learn more about the teachings visit "Abraham-Hicks Publications." Home of Abraham-Hicks Law of Attraction—It All Started Here! Accessed January 14, 2018. http://www.abraham-hicks.com/lawofattractionsource/index.php?i=4.

wow!!!

we can catch excellence." I believe that! I believe that excellence comes with commitment and honesty and follow through, even when you don't think you have an ounce of energy left to succeed. Excellence comes from creating a clean slate with a pure heart and simply accepting that past failures happened, but never letting them define or defeat you. Excellence is then always putting your best foot forward knowing that some days you will just trip and end up with mud on your face, and excellence is always being loving, kind, and good to others, no matter how you may be feeling yourself.

In excellence, you start to choose healthy and nutritionally packed food because it is our friend; food is our healer. It is what tells us every day we put something in our mouths, "I love you back." Your body is your temple. You do need to treat it better, one little step at a time, and it will reward you in return. This I can say and prove to you scientifically. One of my studies examined the mood enhancement of protein pacing with and without physical exercise. It was real. It was definable and thereby achievable for all of you.

I do not want to end part 1 without helping you understand that the key to peak performance, the key to making it to your peak, is by pacing yourself and creating balance in all you do. You can't do it all in a day. It might take many days, it might take longer depending on how committed you are, but the goal is not to just hit the peak and then fall apart and slide down to where you were, like what happens on all diets at some point or another. The key is to constantly be able to remain at your peak, which invariably will change as you age, but doesn't have to be—what you are often led to believe—a life of medicines, failing health, early death, or even feeling like you are held hostage to strict guidelines and restrictive or extreme behaviors, such as counting every calorie and exercising to exhaustion every day. Just the opposite.

The goal of my lifestyle strategies are to provide you time-efficient, sustainable, easy-to-follow, and scientifically proven methods to free you from the shackles that have held you captive with other diets and exercise programs. Visualize daily having a long and healthy life and the laws of attraction or spiritual commitments or positive thinking will bring that energy your way. Pacing is a concept I've come to appreciate more and more and transcends every part of our being, including our relationships, physical nourishment with exercise and nutrition, and our emotional/spiritual well-being. For example, my research shows that consuming the right type and amount of protein at the right time produces the greatest health and physical performance benefit than consuming the same amount of protein less often or not enough protein. Pacing is also critical in our relationships. Science shows the quality of our relationships is significantly enhanced when we take the time to be present with another person, even if it's only a few minutes at a time versus spending an extended period of time with someone but not being present. This is pacing. And the same goes for the time we spend in emotional/spiritual enlightenment. As part of my PRISE Life Protocol, I've included something called a "body visit," which is a daily mindfulness awareness meditation that includes a breathing exercise and time spent in quiet reflection that may or may not include prayer. Again, "pacing" is what's important to maximize the benefit.

Life energy is power, and it is ignited by metabolism in the body, but it is sparked by a thought in the mind. It creates you. It motivates you. It is what inspires you. If you have ever been coached or in a team sport, you will have been taught many ways to help you get over losses or humps, but the one I stand by the most is to train hard (healthy-hard as you learn in part 3, not overexertion hard), but *believe* harder. This is not about "peaking" early. This is not about showing off to others, this is about peaking steadily, enjoying your life along the way, and inspiring others to do the same! As I stated earlier, it's not how fast you start but how long you last. Balance.

Most people may be surprised to learn that, to this day, I am a competitive athlete and a dually certified yoga instructor. Yes, all 6'1/2" of me—coming from a hockey and tennis background, father of three boys from a wonderful wife, Karen—does *yoga*. I know, guys, I might have lost you for a second, so for you, I will call it *stretching*. But the bottom line, this is definitely one of the best practices to keep your body pliable, stretched, and to keep your mind focused. After all, yogis have been practicing this for thousands of years!

I am not naïve. I assure you I have seen a lot and been knocked down my fair share of times. I know that there are many, many obstacles out there. For example, how do I eat at a party or on a holiday? How do I exercise when I work eighteen hours a day? How do I exercise when no one is encouraging me? How do I get off the couch when I have no energy? Obstacles are going to be there every day, but you don't have to bring energy to them. You start with your mind overcoming them, changing and morphing them to positive thoughts, standing up at your computer, walking around, stepping outside, doing some qi gong, putting your bare feet on the ground—every moment that you distract yourself from the negative and move to the positive you have won. And, I know, just by the fact that you have made it to this sentence, every part of your being is becoming a winner now.

You are a winner despite, or better yet, *because* of all your failures, and right now you are going to absolutely let go of comparing yourself to others and what others may or may not have. You can't go through life jealous, hurt, or in fear. All those emotions do is bring your body down and confuse your cells. You will be amazed how the minute you do this, any imagined lack will disappear from your life completely and abundance and gratitude will take over. That is a life to love; that is a sign of peaking daily and staying there! The key is you have to keep your head in the game. You just have to and you can!

Keeping your head in the game means choosing to feel well and not to accept illness, not to allow weight gain or negativity to control you. You can be well, if you choose to. The fact is that we have the fundamental decision-making when we are faced with a healthy or unhealthy lifestyle choice at any given time during the day. For example, do we make the instant choice during the day to eat a healthy snack, such as a banana with peanut butter or carrots and hummus, or do we choose instead, to eat the donut or bagel with cream cheese? Or how about whether to stand up from our chair or couch every hour and take a brisk five- to ten-minute walk around the house, office building, neighborhood, or parking lot instead of choosing to sit and grab another bag of chips, candy bar, coffee or soda as we sit in front of the TV or computer? Sound familiar?

The beginning point of any new healthy lifestyle lies in our heads, our daily life decisions to choose the healthy lifestyle alternative over the unhealthy one. It means showing yourself self-care. I have a quote I wrote because it says it all. "The best health care is self-care. The best self-care is the food we eat, the exercise we do, and the spiritual mindfulness we practice. That's why I developed the PRISE Protocol." *Self-care,* because it suggests the greatest resource to improve our health, resides within each of us. Maybe you have heard the saying, "Physician, heal thyself?" Unfortunately, many of us, myself included at times, ask ourselves why it's even important to choose to be well in the first place? Of course, there are the obvious and well-known health reasons such as, reduced risk for obesity, heart disease, diabetes, cancer, cognitive decline, and mental illness, among others. However, perhaps even more powerful and personal are the subjective reasons, including, clearer thinking, enhanced mental and emotional well-being, greater productivity at work and home, and more physical energy to spend time playing with kids, grandkids, and loved ones.

Sadly, despite all of these real good reasons to be well, we still find lots of excuses not to be well, such as, too tired, not enough time, too busy, don't like to exercise, healthy food doesn't taste good, and the list goes on. While some of these excuses may be true some of the time, many of us use them all of the time. Think about it. From the time the alarm clock goes off in the morning the rat race cranks into full gear, and we drag ourselves out of bed and into the shower to get ready for work. If kids are in the picture, we have the added task (sometimes burden) of trying to pry them up out of bed so they can get ready for the day. Then, we turn our attention immediately to multitasking, which includes grabbing some breakfast, making lunches, and coordinating everyone's schedule before we head out the door for a full day of work! At the end of the work day, of course, it begins all over again—only to repeat itself the following day. Thus, it's no surprise we often choose not to be well. But this is where we need to take charge of our minds, get our heads in the game, and really think about what we may or may not be doing to sabotage ourselves. After all, what excuse do we really have *not* to get well?

I have to share a personal story that completely changed my perspective. For me, the spark to choose to be well was ignited on a cold, wintry morning in 1983 at a health club in Connecticut between classes my junior year in college and during my first week on the job as a fitness instructor. My supervisor asked me to train a young woman scheduled for a training session. I figured, if I was an exercise science major in college and an athlete, I was prepared for just about anyone who walked into the gym. As I turned to meet Tina, she was not walking but being pushed into the gym in her wheelchair. She had cerebral palsy and was nineteen years old, the same age as me at the time.

For the next hour, with me leading Tina through an exercise program, with the help of my supervisor when needed, I was transformed—my spark was lit. I still remember sitting in my cold car in the gym parking lot for several long minutes that day reflecting on how powerful of an experience it was to witness firsthand. Tina, in her compromised physical condition, pushed herself to her limit and seemingly enjoyed the workout with me. As my eyes welled up with tears, all I could think about was how strong her resolve and desire was "to be well" and healthy. In fact, it was right then and there, in my cold, beat-up Ford Escort that I decided to devote my life mission to helping others experience the same opportunity to be well that I shared with Tina on that blustery, cold day. In truth, it was a life-changing epiphany and made me realize that sharing health and wellness with others is contagious, and it's a two-way street. I learned just as much, if not more, about being well and healthy from Tina as she learned from me that day, and I continue to learn and grow from the many students, athletes, research study participants, and clients that I work with on how to achieve optimal health and wellness.

My point to you is, find something or someone that reminds you that you really can do this and that you really should drop the excuses! There is someone you know who is overcoming insurmountable problems and probably hasn't ever had a complaint! Personally, my challenge to myself every day is that I choose to be well so that I may give back to others more fully, the same way Tina gave to me.

Listen, I do understand that there are times in our lives that our minds are our own worst enemy or that we just can't find that spark in life. It happens. It happens to all of us at some point or another. You are certainly not alone. But it is at this moment that, whether you realize it or not, life is offering up a juncture in your life. A chance to overcome and succeed, or a chance to curl up and retreat. Sometimes you need resting time to retreat, so please don't get me wrong, but if you have this book in your hand, there is a glimpse, a hint, a desire to want to tackle the problem and finally get healthy! It is the universe telling you, *it is time*!

While writing this, I want to share that we are *all* constantly evolving, going through those stages of development I spoke about in the first chapter. I'm still going through them myself and, yes, even I am still learning! That is a wonderful thing; ironically it means you aren't dead yet. Recently, I came upon a program, an intensive course called Quantum Emergence, and it's all about discovering the triggers of our emotions and how the pain and suffering we experience in our lives has shaped us. We often refer to this as our "conditioning." If you are truly stuck (meaning you have no idea why you are not getting what you want), can't commit to a plan, can't get your head in the game, perhaps consider taking a look at your conditioning and "beliefs" and how they affect your "emotions."

Unfortunately, the strongest psychological human drive is to behave consistently with the belief we have about ourselves, which perpetuates the same old behaviors over and over again—mind you, not good behaviors! This drive is *faulty* and not accurate and is rooted in the subconscious that relies on early life experiences that originally caused those same emotions, feelings, and reactions. Why are we still repeating them? Because we have forgotten our core. We have forgotten that our true identity is our God-given virtue. Remember how, in chapter 1, I talked about physical strengths and weaknesses that are part of our "nature"? Well, we all have a *virtue*, whether it is faith, valor, perseverance, kindness, and the list goes on, but we can't honor it if we never break through to find out what our calling, our virtue, really is.

In a recent "virtue" reveal, I discovered my virtue, my truth, my identity, is kindness.[32] Defined further, it is "attraction and fellowship and a sense of being appreciated and standing for equality!"[33] All of a sudden, it makes sense that I am a middle child because who else would be the fulcrum in the middle trying to stand there unnoticed waiting to see which side of the teeter-totter will go up or down? Who else has devoted a life to making sure people get the truth no matter the state they are in when they arrive, like Tina? And, may I honestly share, not everyone feels the pride and overwhelming emotion I feel when I am appreciated by an audience or my subjects or my family. It is a feeling I can't explain, but it often brings me to tears. It is in recognizing that early childhood forms the basis of our belief system and, more times than not, they are false and inaccurate. We must go more deeply into our life experiences and understand that once we can target, explore, and realize these original events, we can finally be allowed to overcome our obstacles and our emotions and move into our true being, identity, and calling. It is this truth and so many others that I want you to embrace so that you have a chance to succeed and prosper. You are valuable. Your life has meaning, and it is time to honor every part of you, releasing the old

---

32 "Kindness": A sense of being appreciated and standing for equality. According to the Quantum Emergence System | Dr Matt Mannino. Accessed March 3, 2018. http://quantumemergence.com/qe/.
33 Ibid.

and embracing the new.

The clearer and more focused you can become—remember, eye on the prize—the more amazing the things are that happen. All of a sudden, your path seems to make more sense, and your direction and purpose becomes clear. Instead of fighting yourself every step of the way, you start to actually trust yourself and your decisions. You aren't as hurt by others around you, and you can spend more time in that self-care mode I was talking about. You no longer need to be the martyr or the bully, the over-giver or the taker; you can find balance. And, even more phenomenal, when you find that balance something miraculous happens, something called *second nature* steps in!

Have you ever taken a piano lesson as a child and years later your hands can play the songs, but you don't even know if you can still read music? Or you drive home and don't remember the way, but you get there safely thousands of times? Or you pick up a tennis racquet after you haven't hit a ball in years and are shocked that you can still rally the ball? All of those things are second nature. It's automatic and can save you when you have learned something the proper way, but it can also destroy if it is a bad pattern that you have learned—whether emotional or physical, so be aware.

Second nature is one of the things you are coached on as you become a top athlete—champion—that after you have carefully practiced the skill you are to let go and let your body do the work without fighting it. Experts refer to this as "Mind 1" and "Mind 2." Mind 1 is the critic and judge and always analyzes everything we do, whereas Mind 2 just lets us "be" without any judging or criticizing. It's with Mind 2 that we can reach our full potential and achieve peak performance.

There is a fascinating book I've been reading entitled *Trying Not to Try: The Art and Science of Spontaneity* by Edward Slingerland. I joke because I am a true believer in hard work; however, as I get a little older and wiser, I am much more about working smarter! And no matter your age, it's better to learn this at an earlier stage because it will help keep you from early unnecessary strains, injuries, and overexertion on the body. In this book, Asian Studies professor Slingerland, shares his concept of Wu-Wei (OOO-WAY) and DE (DUH), which deals with spontaneity to foster peak performance. The Wu-Wei is really intriguing because it frees up our minds and allows us to achieve optimal health and peak performance without punishing our bodies by being held hostage and suffering. He teaches how to use spontaneity and effortless flow so exercise and performance can become natural without needing conscious thought. This is how the best performers operate at their peak of performance. The exciting and amazing part is that this is exactly what I did when I created the PRISE Protocol. I made it easy to follow, easy to understand. I brought diversity to it so you never get bored, and I achieved my goal of making it second nature so that you don't have to think about it or use conscious thought and effortful striving, but instead follow the strategies by just doing. The point is that in order to truly reach your peak, and stay there, it needs to become a process that is second nature to you for it to become a permanent lifestyle protocol. Because of this, I am all for discovering anything that may be holding you back and finding a good coach, physically or psychologically, to get you through if you need help.

What did I say in the beginning when I quoted Muhammad Ali? "Champions aren't made in the gyms. Champions are made from something they have deep inside them—a desire, a dream, a vision." I want you to reach down deep and start to really think about that. Think about what you love, what you are afraid of, sports you've dreamed of trying but may have been too scared, things you want to achieve, and ways to remove all the obstacles. I want you to know that optimal health is in your future. I have created something for everyone. You have that champion in you; you only have to decide that you want to seek and then go find him or her.

Jimmy Johnson, the NFL coach, said, "Treat a person as he is, and he will remain as he is. Treat him as he could be and he will become what he should be." I am telling you, in no uncertain terms that you are a champion. You deserve champion treatment. It could be in your relationships, your work, your writings, your art, your athletic abilities, your Tai Chi, your yoga, I don't care what, but *you* have to believe, you have to *know*, you are the champion. You have to know that you do champion your body by your thoughts, and so today I want you to give yourself a talk, a hug, some self-love, and tell yourself and your soul that regardless of what you see in the mirror or in the blood tests or in the past negative news you have had medically that these so-called facts do not control you. You control you. You are the final champion, and you know you are the best. You will win every day you try. You will win every day you eat better. You will win every day you stand up and get outside in nature. You will win every day you set your mind right by getting rid of negative thoughts. You will win every day that your spirit is asked to help, and it picks you up off the floor of desperation to make it the best day of your life. Your heart will fill so full of gratitude, love for yourself, and others that success will be steps away, days away, not months, not years, but now.

And when, or if, you think you are having a bad day, know that you are *my* champion and that if you pull out the little statements and encouragements and truths in this book, they will pull you up and out to become the winner you deserve to be every… single… solitary moment of your life. So, come on! Aren't you ready to follow every protocol in this book and to join me at the peak?

Remember this. Hold on to this. This is the only perfection there is, the perfection of helping others. This is the only thing we can do that has any lasting meaning. This is why we're here. To make each other feel safe.
—Andre Agassi, Open

Let's do this. Get that champion desire on, that vision clear in your head. Let's go out together and serve up a little success each and every day!

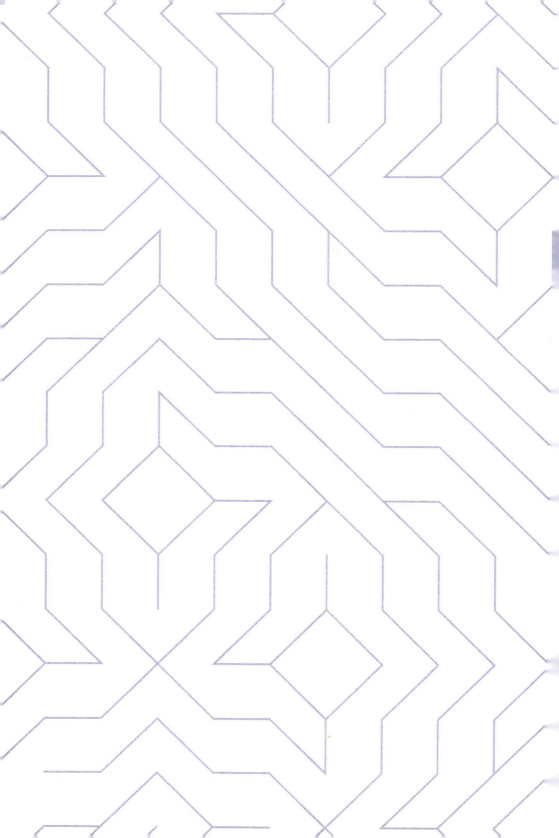

PART TWO

PROTEIN IS POWER AND PACING IS KEY

6

Human Metabolism 101

While weight loss is important, what's more important is the quality of food you put in your body—food is information that quickly changes your metabolism and genes.
—Mark Hyman

It is amazing to me that they don't teach Human Metabolism 101 as early as middle school, because how our body functions should be a necessary course in how to live, eat, and survive. This is one of the reasons I've made it a point to visit elementary, middle, and high schools throughout my thirty-year career and help educate young people on metabolism and the benefits of healthy eating and proper fitness. I even made the news for going to Washington DC and Capitol Hill to speak directly to legislators about the importance of "funding from the National Institute of Health for Heart Disease Research and Stroke Prevention; and then for the school lunch program as well ... making sure that we have adequate funding and programs in place so that our children are fed healthy while at school."[34,35] It was an exciting and eye-opening trip!

I am aware that lots of health books and quick-fix diet books talk about metabolism, healthy eating, and proper fitness, but my goal is to not only refresh

34 "Skidmore professor headed to Washington to talk about health," NEWS10 ABC, May 11, 2015. Accessed March 10, 2018, http://news10.com/2015/05/10/skidmore-professor-headed-to-washington-to-talk-about-health/.

35 The following are a few other newsworthy clips on my commitment to eating healthy, school lunches, and educating children early:

   Salvi, Kristin. "Paul Arciero, New York." You're the Cure. Accessed March 10, 2018, https://www.yourethecure.org/paul_arciero_new_york.

   "Skidmore and local school students mark National Eating Healthy Day." *The Saratogian.* November 07, 2012. Accessed March 10, 2018, http://www.saratogian.com/article/ST/20121107/NEWS/311079911.

   Jennie Grey "Students in Saratoga Springs high school's new nutrition class tour Skidmore College labs." *The Saratogian.* October 22, 2012. Accessed March 10, 2018. http://www.saratogian.com/article/ST/20121022/NEWS/310229936.

your memory but continue to help you debunk some of the latest and craziest theories or misinformation out there. My research has even been touted for its effectiveness in Fox News "Lifestyle," with an article entitled, "How to get into the best shape of your life, according to science!" [36] Another exciting moment in my career! So, when I say after all these years, I've studied and researched what I share, I certainly mean it and can prove it! There is no guessing in my protocols and advice. Let's dive in!

As complex of a biochemical process as the human metabolism is, quite simply its job is to convert food into energy so your body can function. It is much more than just gaining or losing weight as some "experts" have led you to believe. It is sometimes referred to as the engine that keeps us going. It's simple to understand with a car, that you can't put sugar in a gas engine because it kills it, permanently. Well, the food we put into our bodies, for our metabolism engine, determines how fast we can run, how far we can run, and how long we can last. We are living beings that need actual nutrients, from the *food* we eat, to convert into energy, or we, as well, simply stop functioning and get sick or die.

Other than converting food into energy, in the general sense, metabolism also performs another vital role in our lives. This often-missed function is the reason why while some are following a calorie-restricted diet—maybe even pushing their bodies too strenuously with exercise—are still not losing the weight. That other important role of metabolism is aiding the digestive process so that it can actually assimilate nutrients into cells and break down harmful substances. Daily we are faced with poisons, contaminates, toxins, pesticides, drugs, and even alcohol, and these damaging substances need to be removed from the body to survive. This is what I mean when we discuss how important it is to not only nourish our body with proper foods, but conversely, we need to "clean house" and restore the body by releasing these toxins we encounter every day. This is essential for our cells to help our bodies have a shot at functioning optimally for us.

Along with assimilating nutrients (preferably from dirty eating, whole foods, and cleansing with intermittent fasting) and releasing toxins is the important role of using specific proteins properly to control the chemical reactions of the metabolic process. Each chemical reaction is coordinated within the body

---

36   "How to get into the best shape of your life, according to science." Fox News. Accessed March 10, 2018, http://www.foxnews.com/lifestyle/2017/04/06/how-to-get-into-best-shape-your-life-according-to-science.html.

to control other important bodily functions. For example, there are various hormones produced by certain organs (endocrine system) that control the rate at which we can metabolize food, and the reason that if you study a certain group, such as postmenopausal women or individuals suffering from adrenal fatigue, you may find they have other hidden issues. The process of losing weight or gaining health gets a little more complicated because even with the proper and healthy foods, an individual may find they just can't seem to get that scale to budge or their energy to increase. This is where my holistic and integrative approach using my PRISE Protocol, by combining Protein Pacing with my RISE fitness program, has the potential to unlock the magic within each of us, even those struggling with menopause.

Today, you hear so much more about women who are affected with certain illnesses, like that of the thyroid, because thyroxine, one of many bodily hormones produced and released by the thyroid, plays a key role in determining how quickly or slowly the chemical reactions of metabolic process occur within the body. Cortisol is another hormone on the rise and plaguing our society. It's released from the adrenal glands in response to stress (think fight-or-flight response), which also causes sugar (glucose) to be released from the liver. Unfortunately, the more often we are exposed to stress and higher cortisol levels, the more our cells are exposed to higher blood sugar levels and become less sensitive to the hormone insulin. Insulin's primary role is to help shuttle glucose into our cells (muscle and fat), so when it's not doing its job well, blood sugar levels continue to rise and much of the excess sugar finds its way to our belly fat for storage. Thyroids, the endocrine system, and our hormones are all being damaged by the harmful toxins around us such as polychlorinated biphenyls (PCBs), dioxins[37], and dichloro-diphenyl-trichloroethane (DDT)—that first of its kind synthetic insecticide introduced in the 1940s.

Despite this, I have good news. Once you start following my protocol, your body will understand that it is healing. As the confused signals start to clear up

---

[37] "Dioxins refer to a group of toxic chemical compounds that share certain chemical structures and biological characteristics. Several hundred of these chemicals exist and are members of three closely related families: Chlorinated dibenzo-p-dioxins (CDDs), Chlorinated dibenzofurans (CDFs) and certain polychlorinated biphenyls (PCBs). CDDs and CDFs are not created intentionally, but are produced as a result of human activities like the backyard burning of trash. Natural processes like forest fires also produce CDDs and CDFs. PCBs are manufactured products, but they are no longer produced in the United States." "Learn about Dioxin." EPA. March 22, 2017. Accessed February 25, 2018. https://www.epa.gov/dioxin/learn-about-dioxin.

and redirect the internal conversations, with the aid of the beautiful energy from the new food and nutrients you are giving it at the right time, naturally, your body will find the power to produce more energy efficiently. As a result, it will offer you more strength, breathing power, and endurance—more health and life power to enjoy. Who doesn't dream of that?

In expanding your knowledge of chemical reactions and the need for energy to flow, here is the next crucial concept I want you to understand and embrace. It is another natural life cycle that exists perfectly in the human body. You want to think of the body's metabolism as a way to *build up*, *break down*, and *build* itself up again; you may have even heard the terms *anabolism* and *catabolism*. Anabolism, is the *constructive* metabolic process, which is the building and storing function of the metabolism process. It supports the growth of new cells, the maintenance of body tissues, and the storage of energy for future use, so it is the *building up* phase. The second component is catabolism, or the *destructive* breaking-down metabolic process, which is the process that produces the energy required for all activities in the cells. During this phase of the biochemical process—through calories from carbohydrates, fats, and proteins, along with oxygen—it *breaks down* or releases the energy our bodies need to function.

Our bodies are complex but perfectly created, and with proper nutrition, we can help our bodies build up, break down, and build up again. With this concept alone, you will have learned more than most people know. How can we help the process? By carefully thinking about the food we put in our bodies. By carefully picking calories that nourish us versus "empty" or harmful calories, we can actually find that our total energy expenditure doesn't completely deplete us but gives us more hours in the day to feel alert, motivated, and happy.

Empty calories are from foods that provide a lot of calories but have little to no vitamins and minerals and phyto (plant) chemicals. When we are able to consistently nourish ourselves throughout the day with the right amount of nutrient-dense food, at set timing and intervals, we start to see how well we can truly function. It's amazing to think that often that dreaded fat or weight gain is just a sign that your poor body has an energy imbalance, and it is trying to get you to pay attention. It is *conversing* with us, because "food is information that quickly changes your metabolism and genes," as Mark Hyman's quote at the beginning says. The question is, are we listening?

As I've stressed, metabolism is way more complex than the fact that if you consume less calories, then you will lose more weight. Skipping meals or drastically reducing caloric intake to under 500 calories a day regularly, as some diets recommend, is not the wise choice. There is a lot of bad information out there, so beware. When you cut calories that low you are simply forcing your body to go into starvation mode to protect you, and your metabolic process will drastically slow to try to conserve energy and save your life. As a result, it will hold on to every calorie possible giving you the opposite long-term result you are looking for—weight gain, especially fat gain, and with it, the potential to store and hold on to even more toxins!

A body cannot survive without nourishment, and with so few calories consistently, especially without quality calories, it will eventually shut down or starve to death. Don't forget; an obese individual can also starve to death, or a person with pounds and pounds of buildup in decomposing matter stuck in the intestines can starve to death. So again, it goes back to making sure the body can find the time to break down, cleanse, restore, and rebuild itself. Now, be careful here; don't forget what I taught you when I described the difference between the concept of intermittent fasting versus starvation. The first is a "cleaning house" for better health and endurance; the second is depletion so bad you could starve yourself to death or at least become so malnourished that illness will take over. Your stomach will be happy to agree with me on that when it is growling away, because I don't recommend long-term starvation diets!

There are so many fascinating hidden facts about the human body, which is why I have invested all these years researching and teaching. Did you know that even when your body is at rest, it requires energy for the fundamentals, like fuel for organs, breathing, circulating blood, allowing the heart to contract, adjusting bodily hormone levels, plus growing and repairing cells? This is known as the basal metabolic rate or BMR and is the rate of energy consumed by the body at rest. Much of my early research as a nutrition and exercise scientist studied the BMR or more current term, resting metabolic rate (RMR), and I soon became known as the "Metabolism Doctor." To this day, I remain humbled and honored to have contributed much of our current understanding of metabolism based on my scientific research findings in women and men of varying ages, health status, and fitness levels.[38]

---

38   P. J. Arciero. "Resting metabolic rate is lower in women than in men." *Journal of Applied Physiology* 75, no. 6 (1993): 2514–520. doi:10.1152/jappl.1993.75.6.2514.

The RMR is the energy that is just sufficient enough for the function of the body's tissues and vital organs. Believe it or not, usually, a person's RMR is the largest portion of energy use, representing two-thirds to three-quarters of the calories used every day. In most cases, your body's energy requirement to process food remains relatively steady, but I'm going to share with you my proven eating method that can readjust your metabolism in response to eating food at a higher level, so once I help you set the core, you will know what to do to gain or lose weight and even get into peak shape.

As an expert in metabolism, I want to briefly explain the major components of our overall metabolism so you have a much clearer picture of how moment-by-moment lifestyle strategies may greatly benefit our health and fitness. And my PRISE Protocol along with Protein Pacing are the most scientifically effective ways to do this. As I mention above, the greatest contribution of our total daily metabolism, often referred to as our total daily energy expenditure (TDEE) is our RMR because it accounts for roughly 60%–75% of the total number of calories we burn over the course of a day. For example, if you burn 2400 calories a day, your RMR would burn 1440 calories (which is exactly 1 calorie burned per minute over a twenty-four-hour period—there are 1440 minutes in a day) to as much as 1800 calories. The remainder of the calories you burn during the day are the result of three primary metabolic processes:

1) The calories we burn after we eat a meal, also called the thermic effect of food (TEF), accounts for approximately 10% of our TDEE. In this example using 2400 calories a day for our TDEE, it would be 240 calories for digestion, absorption, transport, metabolism, storage, and excretion of food. As I will discuss later, this can change drastically based on the macronutrients (fats, carbohydrates, and proteins) and other foods/drinks we eat and when we eat them.

2) The calories we burn due to physical activity and exercise is called the thermic effect of activity (TEA). This is the most variable, as you can imagine. But for most of us, it ranges from 15%–30% of our TDEE, which would be 360–720 calories a day. This is equivalent to thirty to ninety minutes of walking, jogging, or running a day.

3) The calories we burn while we are NOT sleeping, eating, and exercising are what we refer to as non-exercise activity thermogenesis or NEAT. This could include walking to and from work, parking lot to shopping mall or a friend's house, gardening, working at a computer or other device, and all forms of fidgeting or non-purposeful movements we routinely engage in during the day we may not even be aware of. This may include moving from a seated position to standing for many of us. Or, if you are like me when I'm driving, I constantly shake my legs, which drives my wife bonkers! And our older son, who is a drummer, will often "air drum" while watching TV or sitting in the back seat of the car. This is all NEAT. Amazingly, NEAT can account for as little as 5% to as much as 50% or more of TDEE! That's an enormous range of calories across a day, which can make huge impacts on health and physical performance. In our example, it's 120–1200 calories![39]

Total Daily Energy Expenditure (Metabolism)

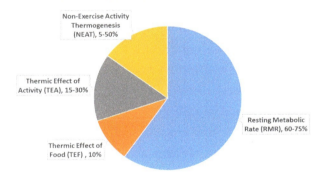

Non-Exercise Activity Thermogenesis (NEAT), 5-50%

Thermic Effect of Activity (TEA), 15-30%

Resting Metabolic Rate (RMR), 60-75%

Thermic Effect of Food (TEF), 10%

My main point to explain this level of metabolism detail to all of you is to show how making small daily lifestyle changes using my PRISE Protocol and Protein Pacing plan can impact your overall metabolism and, more importantly, health and performance in major ways.

While most have heard, and it is true, males do typically have a higher RMR than females. Men have a tendency to have a greater percentage of lean body mass than females of the same age, but don't let that defer any woman reading

---

39   James A. Levine, "Non-exercise activity thermogenesis (NEAT)." Best Practice & Research Clinical Endocrinology & Metabolism 16, no. 4 (2002): 679-702. doi:10.1053/beem.2002.0227.

this book. The great news is that my studies showed incredible weight loss results for both men and women, and neither group felt as hungry all the time![40] Can you see how that alone is a "win" for any lifestyle program? So, although it is true that women tend to have lower levels of lean muscle mass and a higher proportion of fat cells, which, unfortunately, do have a lower metabolism rate than lean muscle mass cells, and they do experience different issues because of pregnancy or later menopause, I am telling you with total confidence and scientific proof that a healthy weight and body composition can still be attained no matter your chromosomes!

Over the years, I've studied so many environmental and lifestyle factors that impact our metabolism, and one of the most powerful agents is caffeine. It's the most widely consumed drug in the world, and the intake of caffeine continues to grow in popularity. What's so fascinating is caffeine has powerful effects on both our central (brain) and peripheral (muscles, fat, vital organs, etc.) nervous system so it's magnitude of effect is vast.[41] On top of that, caffeine is capable of both direct and indirect effects on the body. What this means is caffeine has direct entry into the cells to exert an effect, and it can influence the levels of other substances (hormones, enzymes, etc.) to cause an indirect effect. So, given its widespread impact on our bodies, I took a very comprehensive and integrative approach with my scientific research studies by examining multiple systems and potential effects in both younger and older women and men. Specifically, I conducted two large-scale, intensive research studies examining the metabolic, cardiovascular, and emotional/mood effects of caffeine in both women and men of varying ages. My findings were so impressive, *The Wall Street Journal, Men's Journal,* and other media outlets highlighted them.[42]

---

40 P. J. Arciero, et al. "Resting metabolic rate is lower in women than in men." *Journal of Applied Physiology* 75, no. 6 (1993): 2514–520. doi:10.1152/jappl.1993.75.6.2514.

41 Arciero, P. J., et al. "Effects of caffeine ingestion on NE kinetics, fat oxidation, and energy expenditure in younger and older men." *American Journal of Physiology-Endocrinology and Metabolism* 268, no. 6 (1995). doi:10.1152/ajpendo.1995.268.6.e1192.

42 Additional traditional media sources impressed by my "caffeine" findings:
    Amanda MacMillan, "Why Athletes Should Use Caffeine Patches." Outside Online. April 12, 2017. Accessed March 10, 2018. https://www.outsideonline.com/1786291/are-caffeine-patches-safe-athletes.
    "Laird Hamilton's Bulletproof Coffee Breakfast Recipe." *Men's Journal.* December 05, 2017. Accessed March 10, 2018. https://www.mensjournal.com/health-fitness/bulletproof-coffee-the-new-power-breakfast-20141117/.
    "You Can Now Snort Chocolate, but Doctors Aren't Happy About It." Health.com. Accessed March 10, 2018. http://www.health.com/nutrition/snortable-chocolate-coco-loko.
    "Miracle tricks to burning calories." IOL Lifestyle. November 13, 2016. Accessed March 10,

Here's what I found regarding caffeine's effects on each system. In older and younger women, caffeine drastically increases the amount of calories burned at rest; I call this the thermic response to caffeine. But older women burn half as many calories as younger women, and the amount of fat (fatty acids) appearing in the bloodstream (with the potential to be burned as energy) is similar between the younger and older women—this is great news! Interestingly, the thermic response to caffeine is positively associated with body weight and waist circumference in younger women, whereas positively related to aerobic fitness in older women. This means caffeine's effects may largely depend on body weight and waist size in younger women, but older women should remain active to get the biggest caffeine boost! Regarding heart health, mood state, and caffeine in women, blood pressure is increased and feelings of depression are decreased in older women following caffeine intake, whereas, in younger women, some interesting findings occurred. For one, feelings of tension and vigor increased, and feelings of fatigue decreased. Second, those who are less physically active are more vulnerable to the blood-pressure-raising effects of caffeine than more active younger women. It should be noted that these findings are limited to moderate consumers of caffeine who abstained for forty-eight hours prior to testing, and who ingested the equivalent of approximately two to three cups of caffeine (~240 mg).[43]

Now for us guys. We respond differently to caffeine than women because we showed that older and younger men show a similar thermogenic response to caffeine ingestion, but younger men release much more fatty acids into the bloodstream compared to older men following caffeine ingestion—this is not so great news for older men. Similar to women, the older men increased blood pressure after caffeine ingestion, but younger men had no change. The mood state changes were fascinating; older men reduced feelings of tension and anger whereas the younger guys reported feeling angrier... uh oh—you young guys

2018. https://www.iol.co.za/lifestyle/health/miracle-tricks-to-burning-calories-623661.

"How to exercise less and get better results." All 4 Women. June 03, 2014. Accessed March 10, 2018. https://www.all4women.co.za/211583/health/how-to-exercise-less-and-get-better-results.

"Guide to Healthy Drinks." www.be-fit.me. Accessed March 10, 2018. http://www.be-fit.me/guide-to-healthy-drinks-411/.

43 Paul J. Arciero, et al. . "Influence of age on the thermic response to caffeine in women." *Metabolism* 49, no. 1 (2000): 101-07. doi:10.1016/s0026-0495(00)90888-6.

need to watch your caffeine intake![44,45]

As a scientist, once we have determined the starting point of the individual's RMR—remember energy expended at rest—we then move into what happens when we add other lifestyle choices, such as caffeine, food, and exercise to the process. The incredible fact about the body is that there are longer-term effects of frequent physical exercise, and they are that you can actually change the RMR. Some scientists have shown an increase in RMR and others a decrease in RMR with exercise training. The reason for this discrepancy is likely due to the level of fitness of the person. For example, highly trained elite athletes may show a decrease in RMR with intense training due to the metabolism slowing down and working more efficiently to conserve the calories for when they are needed the most, which is during their intense training and competition. Whereas, some scientists, myself included, have shown RMR to increase with exercise training in moderately fit people, as a result of building new lean muscle mass, a myriad of factors such as increased overall activity of the heart and blood vessel system, together with some other bodily functions, hormone release, increased body temperature, tissue repair, increased amounts of lean muscle mass, etc. That is great news because once you have created a base calorie level and released the toxins, should you add exercise, you have the chance to consume higher quantities of healthy foods. You read that right! You will be able to eat more! Just in case that is not enough good news, the topper from some of my research is that we did not ask our participants to exercise, and they still *lost* significant weight![46]

The secret? The entire weight loss success was because of eating the right quality and amount of protein at the right time. This is because of nothing other than my Protein Pacing discovery! Now you will have an entirely new interest in learning the value of protein, when to use it, and how much. With that new question in mind and understanding just a little bit about RMR, we can move on to learn that there are actually different *rates* that your body burns *macronutrients*. Those are the things called proteins, fats, and carbs. Understanding the basics will help you for later in part 3 when I finally reveal how to combine all of

44   PJ Arciero, et al. "Relationship of blood pressure, heart rate and behavioral mood state to norepinephrine kinetics in younger and older men following caffeine ingestion." *European Journal of Clinical Nutrition* 52, no. 11 (1998): 805–12. doi:10.1038/sj.ejcn.1600651.

45   Paul J. Arciero and Michael J. Ormsbee. "Relationship of blood pressure, behavioral mood state, and physical activity following caffeine ingestion in younger and older women." *Applied Physiology, Nutrition, and Metabolism* 34, no. 4 (2009): 754-62. doi:10.1139/h09-068.

46   Arciero et al; ; He et al; Zuo et al) can be reviewed in full at www.priseprotocol.com.

this in my PRISE Life Protocol. You won't have to spend another minute figuring this out for yourself! I'm getting excited just knowing that by having read this far, you are getting a unique, science-based, truthful education, and you care enough about yourself to keep plugging away! See, *champion*!

7

The Miracles of Macros:
Proteins, Fats, and Carbs

In the last chapter, I talked about the incredible biochemical process called human metabolism and that, simply, its job is to convert food into energy so your body can function. Now we are going to dig a little deeper and talk about the next miracles. Often the absolute easiest way to understand the topic of *macronutrients* and how each benefit our system is to think of a car. I've already said you don't put diesel (or sugar) in a gas engine because it kills it, just as putting unhealthy processed and prepackaged food into your body as a staple will eventually kill you. So, forgive me with some upcoming analogies, but in keeping the following concepts alive and easily understood, pull in your eight-year-old magical thinking or imaginary dreaming brain and picture your body as a Maserati or a Porsche or that favorite car you dream of owning. I'm dreaming right now! Understand, you already have value to me, which is why I keep educating, but you should be *priceless* to yourself. I want you to commit to treating yourself better than your favorite car starting today!

How exactly do you do that?

If you weren't raised in a scientific household, but do listen to the news, you may be familiar with the terms *proteins*, *fats*, or *carbohydrates* (carbs for short), but you may not realize these all fit in a category that is titled *macro*nutrients. Yes, those are the "macros" people talk about, a term that may have eluded you. Don't worry; it is much simpler than you may fear. *Macro*, the word meaning large, is simply saying that for the human body to function properly and get the energy it needs through metabolism, you need to have *a lot* of these macros, the nutrients, which get fed to the body, because they are essential to live. They are the proteins, the fats, and the carbs, and they are the fuel that feeds us. However, like all fuels, the quality and quantity, the timing and the amount, all count; however, the human body is created perfectly, and each macronutrient has a valuable role to play.

Macronutrients contained within food provide us energy and fuel. I like to qualify the process and refer to metabolism as digestion, absorption, transport, metabolism, and storage of the chemical energy from the food we eat into the main energy source the body uses called adenosine triphosphate (ATP). Once the food has been digested and is ready for absorption, transport, and entry into the cells of the body, we need to package these macronutrients into smaller units. Most of the carbs we eat become known as monosaccharides, the most abundant of which is glucose; fats or lipids become free fatty acids; while proteins travel and are taken up into cells as amino acids. This process is called diet-induced thermogenesis or the thermic effect of food. It specifically refers to the calories our bodies burn to digest, absorb, transport, metabolize, store, and release from the food we eat.

Here's an interesting piece of information for all of you to remember, and why I don't want you to ever be fooled into thinking that all calories are created equal; they are NOT! For example, if we were to eat 100 calories of three different meals that contained only calories of that type of food—fat, carbohydrate, or protein—the fat-containing meal would only release/burn approximately 3 calories (or 3%) for the TEF; carbohydrates 10–12 calories (or 10%–12%); but protein burns up to 30 calories or 30% increase in metabolism after you eat a meal containing primarily protein! This is the exact reason why protein is such a valuable nutrient for our bodies to help with healthy weight control and lean muscle mass. I don't need you to memorize this. There is no test. What's most important is the fact that protein is our metabolism friend because it burns the most calories to digest compared to fat and carbohydrate. Having reviewed that, let's look at each macronutrient a little closer.

I'm going to start with protein because that is the key in my program, and therefore, the very first place to start. The term 'protein' originates from the Greek word *proteios* meaning "primary or first" and is vital to human life. Protein is the major building block in the body, and it builds muscle, connective tissues, and is vital in so many cellbuilding roles. Even skin is built of protein. Protein is our most thermogenic, energy costly (in a good way) nutrient we can eat. What do I mean by energy costly? The beauty of protein is that it takes the body a lot of its own energy to break it down through an "active" process that often takes longer to break it down. Meaning, it requires a lot of energy to process and also triggers certain substances and hormones in the gut to be released and sent to the brain. This is why protein makes the body feel fuller longer than a carbohydrate. The process of using protein properly, in the right amount and at the right time, is what I call Protein Pacing. It is the best strategy to follow to help with weight wellness and peak performance leading to an ideal body composition, especially compared to carbohydrate and even fat overconsumption.

"The building blocks of protein—amino acids—circulate in your bloodstream, portal circulation (liver), lymph system and make up the metabolic amino acid pool."[47] The protein foods we eat have various fates inside the body with almost 40% of the protein being catabolized or broken down and even excreted, and only about 10% of the protein we eat is used by the muscles for protein synthesis and building of new muscle. Proteins are constantly broken down and the component parts used again and again. This turnover rate is variable; some cells in your digestive system turnover in three to four days, while cartilage cells take years to turnover. This variability is important because major organs like the liver and heart will be spared from breakdown during starvation at the expense of not-as-essential cells.[48]

Protein is composed of twenty amino acids, and the great news is if you consume the right amount at the right time, it will help you build healthy, metabolically lean muscle mass and keep your metabolism at a healthy level, which in turn will help you break down and release fat. Other than the fact that protein is essential to create lean muscle mass and repair tissues, when protein breaks down to the nine "essential" and eleven "nonessential" amino acids, it is doing this to keep you healthy and extend your life! I'm always a bit perplexed when other "scientists" or so-called experts downplay the importance of Protein Pacing and instead state that the timing (Protein Pacing) is less important than just making sure you get the recommended amount of protein over a twenty-four-hour period in whatever eating pattern that is suitable or convenient for

---

47   Health A–Z. Accessed March 18, 2018. http://www.betterlifeunlimited.com/healthnews/health_az/is-sues/macronutrients_carbohydrates_proteins_and_fats.aspx.
48   "Recent Perspectives Regarding the Role of Dietary Protein for the Promotion of Muscle Hypertrophy with Resistance Exercise Training." *Nutrients* 10, no. 2 (2018): 180. doi:10.3390/nu10020180.

you. This makes no sense to me. We know, from very good scientific investigations, that our bodies are ideally designed to absorb between 20–40 g of protein per serving. How else can you achieve this if you don't use Protein Pacing? The answer is, you can't. In order to provide the ideal amount of protein for optimal absorption by the gut and to maximally stimulate protein synthesis, the only feasible and logical manner to do this is by Protein Pacing.

It is fascinating to understand the difference between essential and nonessential amino acids, and believe it or not this is where the *right type of food is essential*. The only way the body can get the nine essential amino acids (technically, eight for adults) to live is by the food *we put* in our mouths! Understand how significant this is because you can either build up and support your body with proper use of good protein or you can destroy your body by leaving out some of the essential amino acids. We control this, no one else can, and we must in essence treat it like our favorite car! Therefore, while the "nonessential" amino acids simply mean that the body has a way of creating these internally, it is not quite as important that you get each of them in your body through food. However, it is important that you are eating the *right* sources of food to aid the overall process.

As for storing, "Proteins aren't really stored in the body as an energy source but instead the building blocks of protein, called amino acids, are used as building blocks for nearly every cell in the body. By the nature of its structural function, muscle is the largest 'construction site' in the body that uses protein."[49] On a per volume basis, the brain is actually the largest "consumer or user" of amino acids. Ultimately, Mother Hen, the liver, stores the greatest amount of amino acids as it gets ready to send them to the tissues that need to be repaired, rebuilt, or built new. But since muscle is the primary site for amino acid uptake to support muscle cell growth, this is the way that bodybuilders to fitness and performance achievers use protein to build lean muscle mass and also amp up their RMR.

I don't want you to get too caught up in the details here though, because it could feel overwhelming, so let's just go back to the simple car analogy. Think about proteins as the *frame* of your car. Remember, you only get one frame for one lifetime. How are you going to treat it? Only you can keep it from rusting

---

49   Health A–Z. Accessed March 18, 2018. http://www.betterlifeunlimited.com/healthnews/health_az/issues/macronutrients_carbohydrates_proteins_and_fats.aspx.

year after year, and those nine essential amino acids that you make sure you get from the food, will determine the longevity of the vehicle. Perhaps that will make you think twice about what is going into that body of yours!

Thanks to the media, the fear that may be surfacing as you realize that I am telling you to eat protein and later fat, may be, "Oh, no, now I am definitely going to gain weight!" Not true. It is nearly impossible to gain fat from eating too much protein—one of the most well-known untruths in nutrition. Of all the nutrients, protein in excess is the least likely to be converted to fat. In fact, in our current society, our intake of protein has declined in direct linear proportion to the increase in obesity since the 1970s. And, of all the macros, protein is the least likely to be used by the body to make energy. Its priority is to help build and repair cells and tissues. This is also a major reason why protein is *not* used and stored as an energy source (with the exception of small amounts of Branched Chain Amino Acids during stress, intense exercise, and prolonged starvation). They are too committed to the vital role of building and repairing tissues and cells.

While we are talking misconceptions, some people still believe that protein can only be found in meat and dairy products. This is far from the truth because there are both animal and plant protein sources, and this opens up a whole new way of eating while getting healthy proteins into your body. That's why I shared my thoughts in part 1 on whey, pea protein, etc.

Re-familiarizing yourself with metabolism and macros, and remembering that I am all about the lifestyle changes and not the diets, I want to take a minute to discuss the other high-protein diet misconceptions. Thirty years of nutrition and metabolism research has taught me a valuable lesson: Our bodies thrive on a diet consisting of 25% to 35% lean, healthy protein (from both plant and animal sources), along with at least 25% healthy fats and oils, lots of fresh veggies, certain whole grains, and fruit. I will teach you about the *exact* portion and timing of using protein and the importance of making sure that each of those meals contain a quarter to a third protein later.[50] Yet, even with scientific proof, there are still some non-believers.

Despite my published research, as well as research by others that supports a Protein Pacing plan, a recent article in the *New York Times*, "The Myth

---

50   Arciero et al. Studies listed in Bibliography; specifically 2008; 2013; 2014). (*Am J Clin Nutr*: 2011,93:836-43; 2013;97:848–53).

of High-Protein Diets," written by a well-known cardiologist (Dean Ornish, MD) cites a limited perspective of current dietary intake trends and the obesity epidemic using data from the US Department of Agriculture from the period 1950–2000. In stark contrast, more recent peer-reviewed scientific data paints a much different picture of food intake trends and prevalence of obesity among Americans from the period 1970–2010.[53] While both sets of data agree that food intake increased approximately 200 calories per day during this time period, the source of where those additional calories came from differs drastically.

Ornish places the blame on fat and protein. But the published data clearly shows Americans ballooned after eating too many of the wrong carbohydrates during this time period. In fact, current research data strongly supports that for every 1% increase in calories from protein and 1% reduction in carbohydrate calories, overall food intake may decrease by 33 calories a day! In other words, the more protein you eat, the less total calories you consume, and the more likely you will lose weight and improve your health.

I stand firm and say that protein (and fiber) holds the key to weight loss. Several recent intervention studies from our laboratory provide strong support for eating a Protein Pacing diet—think a quarter to a third of your daily calories to decrease total body weight and body fat (including abdominal fat) while improving cardiovascular and metabolic health. Our study diets range between 25% and 35% high-quality animal and plant-based protein that emphasize foods such as nuts/seeds, legumes, beans, pea/rice protein powder, free-range eggs, grass-fed dairy products (milk, Greek yogurt, cottage cheese, whey protein powder), wild fish, and grass-fed beef.

In a lab, this can be easy to control for, but from a practical standpoint, relying on only plants to meet your daily protein requirement can become a full-time job. For example, sound science has proven four or more protein meals per day containing a minimum of 20 g of protein optimizes protein synthesis, quenches hunger, and stimulates metabolism in people under sixty years of age, all of which helps maintain an ideal body composition. Relying on only plant-based foods to meet this translates to 3½–5½ cups of cooked spinach, 1–2 cups of cooked lentils, or 2½–4½ cups of quinoa per meal. If you add physical activity and exercise to the mix, or an age of sixty and older, you would require even more (up to 40 g of protein per meal).

Wow!

Meat is a vital protein source, and one that should be embraced. The important thing is to shop for meat with the same care many people put into shopping for vegetables: with a focus on quality. Not all animal meat is created equal. It is pretty well-known that differences exist between the quality of animal protein from conventional production facilities where the animals have been grain-fed in feedlots or cages versus free-roaming and pasture/grass-fed. Grass-fed beef has a greater amount of heart-healthy omega 3 fatty acids. This is the case for most animal protein sources, including milk, eggs, pork, and fish. Humanely treated and "in-the-wild" animal sources provide a healthier source of nourishment. This quality of animal protein also supports local farmers, which is great for the community and the environment.

So, I say, get your protein and don't be afraid of it. To summarize, I strongly recommend 25% to 35% lean, healthy protein (from both plant and animal sources), and, again don't worry, because I tell you exactly which ones, what portion, and when to consume them in part 3. Again, think protein is the *frame*; you only get one in a lifetime. What are you going to do to protect it like you would your favorite car?

Let's move on to fats. Between the energy-generating macros of carbs and fats, fats take the longest time to generate ATP (energy) in the body. But the good news, once they are broken down, they provide us twice as much energy as either carbs or protein (9 versus 4 calories per gram). Fats are a highly efficient form of energy because they are stored without much, if any, water, and the body has nearly a limitless storage capacity of fat. One word of caution: the human body is designed to store fat relatively easy, and one way this happens is when we overeat carbs, especially simple carbs. As stated, the most popular sites for fat accumulation are under our skin (subcutaneous fat) and especially around the belly (abdominal fat) and our vital organs (visceral fat)—this is the most harmful. We also deposit fat and cholesterol inside our organs, which is definitely not good because it blocks blood (and oxygen) flow to vital organs (heart and brain). Don't be alarmed. Fats provide us lots of great benefits, such as insulation, energy, protection, hormone production, immune system support, etc. Because we store fats so readily in our bodies, the primary goal is to burn them for fuel every chance we get, especially at rest, while we sleep, and even during physical activity.

In the coming pages, I will tell you exactly how to use the macro called fat, but I want to take this moment to share about the dangers of building up fat, and, of course, where most people "store" it. As a Fellow of the Obesity Society, we continue to monitor research and information, and the sad fact is that as a nation the numbers of people struggling from obesity are increasing at alarming rates. People need to understand that we store fat in our cells and even carry them in the blood in the form of triglycerides. We are all well aware of times we carry too much fat on our bodies once we take our clothes off, with most men storing it in their bellies and women around the hips and thighs—until menopause, then they also store it in the belly region. But what you might not have known is that we also store a large proportion of fat inside our muscles and especially around our internal organs (visceral). It's this internal visceral fat that is the most dangerous and increases our risk for cardiovascular (heart) and metabolic (diabetes) disease and certain cancers.

Much of my research has directly quantified/measured the amounts of the harmful visceral fat before and after following my prescribed nutrition and exercise program; the results have been astounding! Visceral fat is reduced by huge amounts *every* time. This is not a common occurrence with many weight loss and gimmicky diets, so be careful. Oftentimes, many calorie-restricting diets cause weight loss in the form of subcutaneous fat loss and even muscle mass loss without a substantial amount of visceral fat; when this happens, it's disastrous! You won't have to worry about this happening with my protocol. Much of the fat loss occurs in the belly and visceral fat region, and the proportion of lean muscle mass is preserved and even increases! Whoo hooo!

There is one other location we store triglycerides and that is in our muscles. I know it sounds weird, but it's actually pretty fascinating how this works. We call this intramuscular triglyceride (IMTG) storage. Interestingly, people who carry large amounts of body fat, termed obese, and even those who have type 2 diabetes, have larger amounts of IMTG than say normal-weight people. Here's where it gets a bit strange. Endurance-trained athletes have similarly large amounts of IMTG as the obese and type 2 diabetics.[51] However, the effects of this similar amount of IMTG in both groups is vastly different. In the individuals

---

51   Bryan C. Bergman et al., "Intramuscular triglyceride synthesis: importance in muscle lipid partitioning in humans," *American Journal of Physiology-Endocrinology and Metabolism* 314, no. 2 (2018): doi:10.1152/ajpendo.00142.2017.

with greater body fat and type 2 diabetes, this greater IMTG causes an associated disease condition called insulin resistance, whereas the elevated IMTG in
the endurance athletes is linked to the opposite effect called insulin sensitivity,
which is good. We call this the athlete's paradox of IMGT. More importantly is
the reason why this occurs. Our bodies are always trying to work as efficiently
as possible as a highly tuned machine, so knowing that fat holds twice as much
energy (9 versus 4 calories) as protein and carbs, this is a preferred fuel source,
especially for endurance athletes. As a result, the muscles respond very smartly
by storing greater and greater amounts of fat (triglycerides) within the muscle
itself as opposed to always relying on it being delivered by the fat (adipose) cells.
It's a longer transit time, and when you are exercising, time is of the essence. So
being able to store this high-energy fuel source directly in the muscle makes
much more sense. Pretty cool stuff, right? I love how the body is always working
to make us perform at a higher and higher level.

This is exactly why I designed Protein Pacing and the PRISE Protocol.

Now what about the media hype that fat is what makes you fat? Let me clear
that up just like I cleared up that too much protein won't make you fat. Fat has
had a terrible rap over the years with the low-fat craze, but, please understand
that your body needs fat, through good food choices, to protect and nourish
your vital organs like your heart and brain, and it is also essential in the assimila-
tion of certain vitamins.

Here are my thoughts on good and bad fats and where to draw the line.

Fats have been ostracized and treated as the "black sheep" of the food group
beginning with the 1980 US Dietary Guidelines. In the early 80s, I vividly recall
my dad trying to lose a few pounds and coming home from the grocery store
each week with low/no-fat everything—ice cream, milk, cheese, cookies, crackers, yogurt, and even potato chips. Despite eating all of these low/no-fat foods,
he struggled losing those extra pounds. I think many people can relate here.

The most disturbing irony of the low/no-fat diet recommendation is that
the more Americans have avoided eating fat, the fatter we've become as a nation.
The most telling evidence of the growing obesity epidemic is highlighted in the
Centers for Disease Control (CDC) figures beginning in 1985 that track the
obesity epidemic and trends in parallel with the low/no-fat craze.[52] They show

---

52 "Overweight & Obesity." Centers for Disease Control and Prevention. August 31, 2017. Accessed
February 25, 2018. https://www.cdc.gov/obesity/data/prevalence-maps.html.

the alarming fact that the low/no-fat diets are dramatically increasing weight. Yes…the statistics are stunning, but there is much to learn from them.

Interestingly, the driving force behind the low/no-fat craze that swept the nation was the US Department of Agriculture (USDA) and Department of Health and Human Services (HHS). In fact, every five years, the federal government appoints a group of scientists to the Dietary Guidelines for Americans Committee (DGAC) with the goal of proposing updates to the Dietary Guidelines for Americans. Up until recently, the group has emphasized low/no-fat foods.

It's pretty well-known that private interests and industry lobbyists played a major role in the "misguided" food guide pyramids we've all been told to follow since 1980, and the low/no-fat recommendation was the first example of this. Fortunately, for the first time since 1980, the most current 2015 DGAC finally removed an upper limit on total fat intake. In other words, they lifted the ban on total fat intake and opened the door to accepting—even encouraging—dietary fat intake as a healthy part of the diet. The article cited here called "Lift the Ban on Total Dietary Fat" published by the *Journal of the American Medical Association (JAMA)* is worthy of a read.[53] Progress!

The scientific data is clear; we need to *eat fat to burn fat* and *all fat is not the same*. Even the *New York Times Magazine* in 2002 addressed this in an article called, "What if It's All Been a Big Fat Lie?[54] A diet rich in healthy fats, such as nut (walnuts, almonds, macadamia), plant (olive, coconut, avocado, palm), and fish oils are the most nutritious and tasty. Opting for the full-fat version of (organic and local) milk, cheese, Greek yogurt, and cage-free/free-range eggs are usually always better options than the low/no-fat versions; so don't be fooled. And because the "primary function of lipids is to form the membranes of each and every one of the cells of our body—billions and billions of them,"[55] and fats also regulate fluids that pass in and out of our cells as well as make cholesterol,[56]

53 Dariush Mozaffarian, "US Dietary Guidelines and Lifting the Total Dietary Fat Ban." *JAMA*. June 23, 2015. Accessed February 25, 2018. https://jamanetwork.com/journals/jama/article-abstract/2338262?res ultClick=3&redirect=true.

54 Gary Taubes, "What if It's All Been a Big Fat Lie?" *The New York Times*. July 07, 2002. Accessed February 14, 2018. http://www.nytimes.com/2002/07/07/magazine/what-if-it-s-all-been-a-big-fat-lie. html?pagewanted=1.

55 Health A–Z. Accessed March 18, 2018. http://www.betterlifeunlimited.com/healthnews/health_az/is-sues/macronutrients_carbohydrates_proteins_and_fats.aspx.

56 Ibid.

never underestimate the role they play.

I know we've heard so much about how bad cholesterol is for you that we tend to overlook the importance of cholesterol. It works right next to lipids in the cell membranes and makes the membranes rigid and able to hold their shape. There are many more membrane functions thought to be attributed to cholesterol's presence. Just like fat is used for insulation and shock absorption as it protects organs and joints from the trauma of movement, cholesterol is necessary for the body. Because we need it for health reasons, low cholesterol diets are not necessarily good for us, unless you have a genetic variant that leads to excess plaque buildup, in which case you should aim to limit your intake to 200 mg/day. But those with this are very rare in numbers.

One point I think worth stating is that dietary cholesterol from foods like eggs (one egg yolk contains approximately 200 mg) make little impact on the cholesterol levels in your blood. Our daily requirement for cholesterol is approximately 300 mg/day. The less cholesterol you eat in foods the more cholesterol your body produces itself. So, the amount of cholesterol you eat really only affects how much your body has to produce itself. Your liver (who I call Mother Hen) likes to keep the cholesterol amount to 1000mg/day to support body needs. Another extremely beneficial strategy to help lower total and LDL-cholesterol (bad cholesterol) is with plant sterols from nuts, seeds, and legumes, as well as Pantethine[57], a derivative of vitamin B5 and niacin, B3. The sterols reduce the absorption of cholesterol by looking and acting just like cholesterol and therefore block cholesterol from being absorbed by the gut and into the bloodstream. Aim to eat foods containing 1.3 g of plant sterols a day

As I have stressed throughout the book, the quality of the fats is everything. To make it simple, don't eat trans fats. They are bad for you and are found in partially hydrogenated oils to make the substance more solid like margarine or even shortening and certain saturated fats (those that get hard at room temperature and come from conventional feedlot animal products), or vegetable shortenings—both increase blood cholesterol and are linked to heart disease. Certain saturated and trans fat can raise low-density lipoprotein (LDL) cholesterol

---

57   Malkanthi Evans, John Rumberger, Isao Azumano, Joseph Napolitano, Danielle Citrolo, and Toshikazu Kamiya. "Pantethine, a derivative of vitamin B5, favorably alters total, LDL and non-HDL cholesterol in low to moderate cardiovascular risk subjects eligible for statin therapy: a triple-blinded placebo and diet-controlled investigation." *Vascular Health and Risk Management*, 2014, 89. doi:10.2147/vhrm.s57116.

(known as the "bad cholesterol") levels in the blood. High total cholesterol or a high LDL cholesterol level is a leading risk factor for heart disease. Having said all that, the great news is you don't have to be afraid of all fats. As a matter of fact, some are really good for you in the proper proportion. Those are monounsaturated fats like olive oil, which is liquid at room temperature, and can even help lower blood cholesterol levels, and perhaps even polyunsaturated and saturated fats, the oils that come from fish, plant, and vegetable origin and are liquid or soft at room temperature and grass-fed cows, respectively. *Mono* means one, and *poly* means many, and for the scientist in you, it refers to how many hydrogen atoms occur in a molecule, or fundamental unit, of fats and oils, compared with carbon atoms.

The most important fact to walk away with is that good fats don't make you fat; they can even lower blood cholesterol levels and help you maintain energy and a proper weight. So, if they were your car, they are the *oil* that feeds the rest of the engine. If you don't put the right oil, a high-quality oil, in a high-end car or even worse let the oil get empty, your engine will cease to function, forever, and no matter how good the frame may be, the vehicle is *morto*, *caput*, yes, dead. So, please, take another look at fats in foods and do choose to incorporate the healthy ones! I recommend at least 25% healthy fats and oils and up to as much as 70% if you are following the fat-adapted, ketogenic diet.

Finally, we arrive at the truth about those carbs! Carbohydrates can't be ignored. Every part of metabolism has been put in order by the creator for a reason. If you have been part of the no-carb phase, I really want you to start to rethink things a little bit. Don't worry; you already know I am not telling you to do carbs, all vegetables, and no protein, but I want to help you realize why you may be so tired with no quick pick me ups. The wrong carbs, or no carbs to give you quick energy, are probably weighing you down, and therefore, you are resorting to caffeine or other sources of stimulants to try to get through the day.

The fact is the right carbohydrates truly are the main, and first, energy sources for the brain and red blood cells throughout the day. Carbs break down into glucose. You need glucose for the brain to function and for your muscles to function efficiently during the day, and especially while exercising. An interesting point about storing carbohydrates is that, "Glucose and fructose are stored in limited quantities in the body in the form of glycogen. The liver stores about

400 calories of carbohydrate in the form of glucose as glycogen, and the muscles another 1600 calories as glycogen with the blood containing roughly 80–100 calories at any one time. Thus, overall your body attempts to keep a 24-hour supply (about 2000 calories a day) of glycogen so you always have a ready supply of glucose available under normal food-intake conditions."[58]

And as per excess, "Carbohydrate intake is converted to fat by the liver and stored in fat cells. Some fat is made this way every day and is necessary to stretch the energy we get from our food. Only when we chronically overeat does the excess fat that's made begin to show up in our favorite fat depositories."[59] Unfortunately, given our excessively high intake of carbohydrates in our culture on daily basis, especially simple sugars, we accumulate and store a lot of excess fat from overeating simple carbs, much more so than an excess intake of fat or protein. Just to be clear, simple carbs are those that are digested really quickly like the sugar in soda and candy, fruit juices, but also the refined and processed cakes, breads, and pastas. Complex carbs that include fiber digest more slowly, don't play havoc with your blood sugar, and are much more advisable. And as I stated earlier, an excess of carbohydrates, especially the simple ones, are easily converted to fat in the liver and then stored in fat cells (adipose cells).

And now for the fun, debunking part, as I talk about "wonder carbs," and I don't mean Wonder Bread! In recent years, no single food group has been "thrown under the bus" more than carbohydrates. This carb backlash reminds me of the low-fat craze I discussed. I want to remove the "diet clutter" and nutrition misinformation and set the record straight on both fat and carbohydrate intake.

Let's revisit the modern-day "no carb" craze. We've all heard the comments, "Are you a 'carb-lover' or maybe a 'carb-addict'?" Perhaps you're gluten-sensitive, have celiac disease, or you're boycotting all "GMO" carbs. I get it … these are all valid and real reasons to keep an eye on your carb intake and not overindulge. However, none of these are healthy and safe excuses to avoid carbs completely.

Carbohydrates come in many different forms, including vegetables, fruits, legumes (beans and nuts), whole grains, and even dairy. To suggest that a no-carb diet is remotely safe and healthy is dangerous. Our bodies need carbs because they provide energy, healthy fiber, essential nutrients, boost immunity,

---

and give food sweetness. The biggest challenge is choosing carb foods that provide the most nourishment and health benefits, yet also taste good. We love our bread, bagels, pasta, potatoes, rice, and cookies, but these are the main culprits to storing excess body fat, especially belly fat. We all know the benefits of eating fresh vegetables and fruits and the health problems of too many starchy carbs.

What if I told you that you can, "Have your cake and eat it too!" Sounds too good to be true, right? Well, I've had the good fortune to examine all kinds of carb diets in my Human Nutrition and Metabolism Lab. What I've learned from others and discovered in my lab is there are types of carbohydrates known as *resistant starches* (RS) that are super healthy and act a lot like fiber. Because the starch (carbs) is not completely digested, it passes into the large intestine (colon), undergoes fermentation, and forms short-chain fatty acids, such as butyrate, which feeds the good bacteria in the gut. Essentially, RS is a potent prebiotic.

Here are the basic facts. There are four main types of resistant starch:

RS 1—Starch found in beans, seeds, whole grains, and pasta with durum, contains a protein matrix, which hinders its digestibility.
RS 2—Starch found in common foods such as uncooked potatoes and unripe bananas, are resistant to enzyme breakdown until ripening or cooking.
RS 3—Also called retrograded starch, develops in starchy foods after cooking then cooling them (fridge or freezer), resulting in structures that make them resistant to digestion. Commonly occurs in cooked and cooled potatoes, grains (pasta, rice), and beans.
RS 4—Chemically modified resistant starch that doesn't occur naturally and is usually made with "hi-maize resistant starch."

I'm a huge fan of RS 3 foods because they are "leftovers," easy to prepare, and taste really good. Next time you cook potatoes, pasta, rice, or beans, consider preparing them the night before and then refrigerate (cool) and eat the next day. You will create RS and lots of strong, healthy bacteria in your gut.

In my lab, I tested RS 4 starches using a pancake breakfast I fed to women and men on four different visits to my lab. The results were astounding! In the first study, after eating the resistant starch pancakes, *women burned 20% more*

FAT, reported feeling 80% more "full" and 25% less "hungry" compared to traditional pancakes.[60] I encourage you to read my published scientific study to learn about the benefits of eating RS 4. It's very likely the other RS types (1–3) produce similar results. They truly are wonder carbs!

And last but not least, after you figure out the percentage you are sticking to for protein and fat, the remainder will go to carbs. Don't lessen their importance though; those carbs are the gas, the fuel, that keep you going all day long, and as we know, no gas, no go.

With your refreshed memory on macronutrients, I can share a fascinating few additional points. In order to lose fat, the fat molecule needs oxygen and a background level of carbohydrates to complete the chemical breakdown. It is important to ensure your body has an adequate supply of high-quality carbohydrates during your workout. When this carb supply is exhausted, the body struggles in burning fat the way it usually does and instead starts to break down fat in a process called ketosis. In extreme cases of carbohydrate depletion, a person "bonks" and cannot continue performing any type of exercise because the muscles basically stop working.

However, in some cases, the body is able to adapt to this low/no carbohydrate-higher fat state by partially burning body fat stores for energy by producing ketones. Ketones are produced when you've either fasted for a few days or drastically restricted your intake of carbs to less than 100 calories a day. When this happens, fat is not able to be broken down and burned through its normal pathway. The dilemma is when carbs are depleted, the brain and nervous system need another source of energy, but they are not able to use fatty acids.[61]

Fortunately, the brain, organs, and muscles can use ketones as an energy source. Mother Hen comes to the rescue by producing ketones from partially broken down fat. In fact, the liver is so committed to the production of ketones when the carbohydrate supply is depleted that it cannot even use the ketones as an energy source and supplies them all to the rest of the body, especially the brain. If this isn't an example of Mother Hen, then I don't know what is! This

---

60   Christopher L. Gentile, Emery Ward, Jens Juul Holst, Arne Astrup, Michael J. Ormsbee, Scott Connelly, and Paul J. Arciero. "Resistant starch and protein intake enhances fat oxidation and feelings of fullness in lean and overweight/obese women." *Nutrition Journal.* October 29, 2015. Accessed January 20, 2018. https://nutritionj.biomedcentral.com/articles/10.1186/s12937-015-0104-2.

61   For further details read: Anssi H. Manninen, *Journal of the International Society of Sports Nutrition.* 2004. Accessed March 3, 2018. https://www.ncbi.nlm.nih.gov/pmc/articles/PMC2129159/.

is the premise of the ketogenic fat-adapted diet. However, beware, this takes a minimum of two to four weeks for most people to transition into this state, which is called the ketogenic hangover—not fun! Also, there is always the risk that muscle may be used as a source of energy during this time, which is not good, so you *must* make sure you follow my Protein Pacing protocol to avoid this. Our goal should always be to preserve our muscle mass at all times, because muscles provide definition and tone. It's also a source of fat-burning since it burns more calories than fat.

You might be asking, "Wait, I heard you burn carbs for energy when you initially start exercising, so what happens when you are fat-adapted or following a ketogenic diet?" Great question! In a non-fat-adapted or ketogenic state, this is absolutely true. Although it does depend on the intensity at which you exercise and your fitness level. For example, the greater the intensity of the exercise, the more carbs you burn compared to fat. At any given level of submaximal exercise (anything less than maximum effort), the more fit you are, the greater amount of fat you will burn at the beginning of the exercise and throughout the exercise compared to a less fit person. So, there is a huge advantage to getting fit so your body can become a fat-burning machine, both at rest and during submaximal exercise.

When exercising at maximal effort, carbohydrates, along with your other immediate energy source within your muscles, called creatine phosphate, becomes your major energy source regardless of your fitness level. Of course, more trained individuals have greater glycogen (stored carbohydrates) and creatine phosphate stores so they are capable of performing at a maximal effort for longer and at a higher output. Turning back to the ketogenic or fat-adapted state, at the onset of exercise you are already nearly depleted of carbohydrate/glycogen stores, so the body becomes conditioned to initiate exercise using ketones and then to rely on them for the remainder of the exercise bout. This turns the body into a fat-burning machine right from the start. Finally, as briefly mentioned above, you should get your heart up to a certain rate. Once there, you can be sure that your body will ultimately start metabolizing fat.

Another important tip I want to stress is that aerobic, endurance, or submaximal exercise is *not* the best type of exercise to burn and release your fat stores. It's actually my interval training, also called high-intensity interval

Wow!

training (HIIT) or sprint interval training (SIT). I know I just explained that we burn the most fat during submaximal exercise compared to maximal all-out exercise. However, when we perform intervals, the exercise intensity is so high that the extreme demand on the metabolic pathways within our muscle cells causes the enzymes to undergo a change that results in making them more active and responsive and grow in number. This translates into a greater capacity for our cells to utilize oxygen and therefore metabolize fat during both resting and exercise states. In addition, the high intensity of intervals burns a lot of calories and increases your heart rate, body temperature, breathing, hormone levels, blood flow, and muscle contractions, which all increase the "afterburn" or in scientific terms what we call the excess post-exercise oxygen consumption (EPOC) for up to seventy-two hours! Even more amazing, a growing body of scientific evidence clearly shows that doing intervals has the greatest impact on revving up the enzymes responsible for breaking down and burning our body fat energy stores. This should be great news for all of you, because now you don't have to spend hour after hour running/walking/jogging, stepping on the elliptical all day, etc. thinking this is the only way to shed the excess belly fat. As I will describe in the coming chapters, it takes only twenty to thirty minutes once a week of intervals to blast the belly fat!

Don't worry; you can come back and read this later if you are feeling "HIIT" with too much information, but I'm now even debunking "The Myth of the Fat-Burning Zone." You know how every piece of exercise equipment recommends you exercise at a submaximal level within a certain range of your heart rate to maximize your fat burning? This is a total myth. That is *not* the best way to burn body fat. The best way to burn body fat is with intervals to increase the "afterburn" or the EPOC. I do discuss this afterburn and touch on these topics more in part 3.

This leads me to my final point: The other elephant in the room.

I can't end the chapter without touching on the big weight loss *lie* that calorie counting is key. I'm sorry to burst your bubble, but counting calories is *not* the answer to improved health and performance. I know, I know, who do you trust? More than 75% of Americans at any given time are trying to lose or maintain weight, and for good reason. We are one of the most obese (fattest) nations in the world. Unfortunately, the more than $190 billion spent each year on medical expenses to treat obesity-related diseases also proves this fact.

With all these weight-loss strategies, some that are based on scientific research, too many of them are just gimmicks. Nearly all of these weight-loss strategies emphasize "counting calories" by restricting your food intake and/or increasing the amount of exercise and physical activity you perform each day to burn more calories than you ingest. It becomes a "zero sum game" and puts our bodies and minds in constant conflict. This, of course, is where the biggest problem arises for most of us. We love to eat and hate to move! As a result, we are often doomed for failure even before we start a weight-loss program. It's frustrating and exhausting to have to live on a low-calorie diet or exercise to exhaustion every day for hours.

I address the fact that quality eating is top priority and share with you examples in chapter 15. It is less about the quantity of how much you're eating *when* it is quality food that is being ingested! For the record, I never mention weight loss or dieting to my clients, athletes, and research study participants. I am not concerned whether they lose any weight at all, and I do not focus on "how many calories" they are eating or burning with exercise. I avoid a "calorie-counting" mentality and instead encourage nourishment through eating the right types of food and choosing the right types of exercise and activity. If you are nourishing your body throughout the day with the right type, amount, and timing of the most critical and vital nutrients your body needs to function optimally—with the right amount of protein to keep your muscles and cells functioning optimally and signal to the brain that it's satisfied—you will maximize your health and performance and have the energy to add fitness training. I fully understand and appreciate the laws of thermodynamics when it comes to calories in and calories out[62], but lots of really good science support the major role of protein tipping the scale as a superior macro to support optimal body weight and composition. I am all about helping people optimize their overall health, body composition, and physical performance by teaching and

---

62   Please refer to:

S. Howell and R. Kones, "Calories In, Calories Out and Macronutrient Intake: The Hope, Hype, and Science of Calories," *American Journal of Physiology, Endocrinology and Metabolism*, November 01, 2017. Accessed March 26, 2018, https://www.ncbi.nlm.nih.gov/pubmed/28765272.

C. D. Gardner et al., "Effect of Low-Fat vs Low-Carbohydrate Diet on 12-Month Weight Loss in Overweight Adults and the Association with Genotype Pattern or Insulin Secretion: The DIETFITS Randomized Clinical Trial," *JAMA*, February 20, 2018. Accessed March 26, 2018, https://www.ncbi.nlm.nih.gov/pubmed/29466592.

guiding them with scientifically proven lifestyle strategies to achieve their best results and keep them motivated and committed to staying on a healthy path.

When you follow my program, you will have the best side effect ever! You will find it to be an effective strategy to accelerate body fat (especially belly fat) loss; build lean muscle mass; enhance metabolism; lower blood sugar, cholesterol, and blood pressure; release toxins from body fat; and greatly enhance physical performance. There is plenty of excellent scientific research showing that when you favorably change your body composition (without losing any weight) you also significantly enhance your health and physical performance. By following a healthy lifestyle program, such as PRISE—that incorporates scientifically proven strategies that show you how to eat healthier, exercise properly, and reduce stress—you will *not* have to worry about counting calories to lose any weight by starving yourself or exercising every day to exhaustion, but instead learn how to enjoy each day and live your life to the fullest!

With our little refresher course on macronutrients, understanding that quality over quantity, not counting calories, and learning that if we exercise properly, our bodies can even burn fat at rest or during submaximal levels, you are now primed to understand how important each macronutrient is and a little about their true roles. In the end, metabolism and getting the proper macronutrients is all about energy expenditure to give your body life power, and by balancing it is revealing the correct amounts to use when, so you, too, can gain optimal health. Overall, human nutrition and metabolism is evolving so rapidly it's important to have access to the latest scientific research on the health and performance benefits of all different types of food, including proteins, fats, and carbs, as well as immediately dispelling the new myths that seem to be spreading rapidly every day.

I hope this also helps you understand why my research has been validated and embraced worldwide. I don't want you to have a shortened "shelf life" because you ignored the natural life cycles of our food and our bodies, or you didn't pay attention to the value and purpose of macronutrients. I want you to live and eat and find the energy and life source that makes you abundant—that makes you a gift to the universe as you were meant to be. I want your Maserati or Porsche, to last a long, long time.

I know I have discussed a lot, but let me summarize some key points from

2 Ways to Wear...
The 'Coatigan'

ONE PART COAT, ONE PART CARDIGAN, THIS COZY KNIT WORKS WITH EVERYTHING

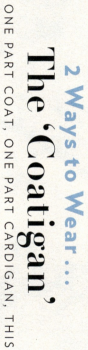

Jennifer Lopez in Max Mara

FOR THE OFFICE

Ann Taylor, $149; anntaylor.com

Exclusive discount! Get 20 percent off this knit with code 'COATIGAN' through 1/27!

Turtleneck
A neutral complements the houndstooth print.
H&M, $18; hm.com

Metallic

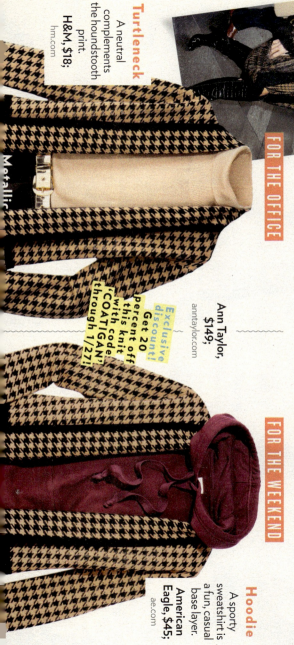

FOR THE WEEKEND

Hoodie
A sporty sweatshirt is a fun, casual base layer.
American Eagle, $45; ae.com

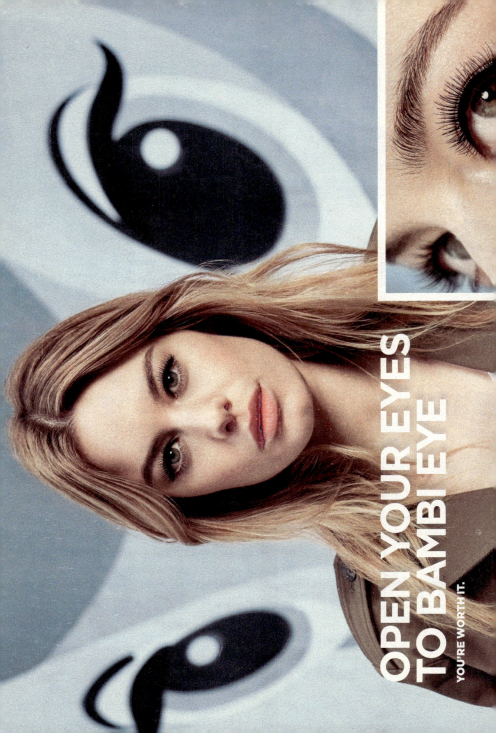

OPEN YOUR EYES
TO BAMBI EYE

YOU'RE WORTH IT.

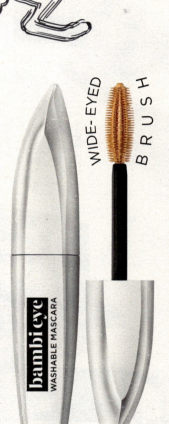

LASHES ENHANCED WITH LASH INSERTS.

©Disney

NEW

bambi eye

MASCARA

INSTANT EYE-OPENING RESULT, VOLUMIZES AND CURLS, LASH BY LASH

WIDE-EYED BRUSH

WASHABLE MASCARA

bambi eye

L'ORÉAL
PARiS

Faux Leather Skirt

The sleek fabric balances out the knits on top. **Universal Standard, $100;** universalstandard.com

Pop on a gold belt for a touch of shine. **Zara, $26;** zara.com

Top Handle Bag

A structured satchel with gold hardware ties it all together. **A New Day, $37;** target.com

Burgundy Booties

Try a stacked heel with a subtle pop of color. **Franco Sarto, $149;** macys.com

Geometric Earrings

Minimalist hoops are simple yet sophisticated. **Kendra Scott, $65;** kendrascott.com

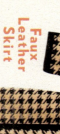

Style Tip!

Give this outfit a more waist-defining shape by half-tucking the sweatshirt.

Relaxed Denim

Update your comfy jeans by rolling them up for a cool cuff. **Gap, $70;** gap.com

Roomy Tote

This lightweight find folds up into a small pouch. **Baggu, $44;** baggu.com

Leather Sneakers

The olive-gray color elevates your basic kicks. **Keds, $90;** keds.com

By **SARAH BALL**

the last few chapters. The longer-than-normal shelf life wreaks havoc on the human body because the harmful chemicals used to protect and stimulate the growth of the vegetable, fruit, grain, or animal gets passed on to the cells in our bodies. Synthetic chemicals contribute to the current plague of modern-day diseases, such as cardiovascular and metabolic disease, certain cancers, as well as inflammatory and neurodegenerative disorders. Macronutrients in the right portion at the right time, especially protein, will make almost any "diet" program you follow a success. Use a discerning eye so that you follow the truth and not the "fake" truth created by media and half-truths.

Once you really assimilate and start trusting these ideas, you will start following my protocol with ease and comfort, and your body will understand that it is healing. The conversations within your cells will multiply and even speed your healing and performance. The beautiful nourishment from the new food and nutrients you are giving it will produce more energy efficiently and, as a result, give you more strength, breathing power, and endurance—more life power to enjoy. That is the power that Mother Nature gave us to use, not abuse.

Will you join me, then, in spreading this message and getting it to others? I asked a question in the very beginning of this book: Will you choose a life that will help others and yourself thrive and find balance or will you continue to destroy the gift of life you have been given? I am giving you the keys. The keys to your priceless car. I am unparalyzing you by providing up-to-date, time-tested material that has already been shared with millions and is having life-saving effects. Isn't it your turn to choose the most incredible life energy around? Remember, protein is power, so now let's learn how pacing is key!

8

Protein Pacing:
The Right Type and Amount
of Protein at the Right Time

Adopt the pace of nature: her secret is patience.
—Ralph Waldo Emerson

You may say, "I have tried every diet or lifestyle change out there, Dr. Paul. Why will this one work?" That is the *point*. You *have* tried every diet out there, and every diet is missing this one piece. With it, you finally have the key ingredient to make even other "healthy diets" work. With your mind-set and motivation renewed from part 1, I want you to not only walk away with a willingness to make a personal change for the better for you and your loved ones, but know that you can and will. You are *the* champion. If you are on a diet or have ever "practiced" or followed a certain diet, it is time to make a change. Your health and body's performance as well as longevity depend on it. No more practicing; it's time to commit. Go back and read the power the mind has and the concepts of "second nature" in chapter 5 if you need motivation again.

In the meantime, to keep you on track, here is a powerful quote that I love:

"Success is never final, failure is never fatal. It's courage that counts."
—John Wooden

Courage! Depending on where you are at with food, nutrition, and exercise, my protocol will either become the quicker-fix key that is missing to your current diet or your awakening to the fact that the answers are here and you can absolutely make these easy changes in your daily routine for dramatic success. No matter what your situation is, this will move you from having been on diets to making the final plunge to a permanent, healthy, invigorating, energizing, and mobilizing lifestyle of healthy eating and reasonable exercise. As I also said in the beginning, there is no risk, no downside to this protocol, and if you follow it as I have set it up, there is *guaranteed scientific* success. Few, if any, other doctors or experts to date can say that.

I've debunked the diet myths, shared information on ethical scientific research, shared some on metabolism and the power of the mind, and now I am putting every step that needs to be followed out there, because no matter how hard you try to convince me otherwise, the fact is that people are still confused on what they should be eating and how they should be exercising. How do I know? For the mere fact that thousands upon thousands of books have been written and people are still obese and confused and sick. The fact that other experts are seeking me out for advice and that millions upon millions are now looking at my research and quoting or following it, only adds to this fact.

So far, we've discussed the deeper benefits and need for protein, but we need to do them at the right time, even if leading nutrition scientists are at odds over which diet is the best for us—they can't argue with the next piece I share!

There is one common denominator among all of these various diets that *all* nutrition and diet experts agree, and I am the nutrition scientist who developed this nutritional strategy. It's Protein Pacing. Because I've established this long career investigating both the acute and longer-term impact of nutrition (meal timing and distribution), exercise (quality vs. quantity), and emotional well-being lifestyle interventions on health and physical performance, I have emphasized the heart health, metabolism, hormonal fluctuations, body composition, brain health, and physical performance outcomes of these interventions on both optimal health and disease risk in women and men across the age and fitness spectrum. It all came down to one major *protein* revelation.

What many consider to be my most important scientific discovery was the observation that consuming ideal amounts (20–40 g per serving) of high-quality protein four to six times per day (with and without exercise training), people reduced total body and abdominal fat to a greater extent than three "traditional" higher-carbohydrate meals per day. This work was published in the

Obesity Journal in 2013 (Impact Factor: 4.3) and *Journal of Applied Physiology* in 2014 (Impact Factor: 3.4) and led to the terms "Protein Pacing" and "PRISE Protocol", as well as numerous additional peer-reviewed publications. In fact, the highly acclaimed monthly medical newsletter "Duke Medicine Health News" published a four-page feature article highlighting my Protein Pacing and PRISE Protocol research. In addition, my Protein Pacing and PRISE Protocol has also been extensively cited in other medical publications such as, the aha. org (American Heart Association "American Heart Association & Dr. Paul"), *Science Daily* and *Villanova COPE*. My protocol has also been cited in mainstream popular media, including: *The Wall Street Journal,* Fox News, *Prevention, Good Housekeeping,* WebMD, *O Magazine, TIME, Huffington Post, Daily Mail, SELF, Glamour, Shape, Health, Women's Health, Women's World, Muscle and Fitness, Men's Fitness, and Men's Health.* Other national media outlets include: "Doctor Radio XM/Sirius," "Guru Performance," and "Rusty Lion Podcast" on iTunes. The National Public Radio program "Academic Minute, Best of Our Knowledge" has not only featured my research but also awarded me the 2015 Most Likely to Change the World Senior Superlative Award. I'm also a member of the International Protein Board, comprised of the top protein scientists in the world (www.internationalproteinboard.org).

With all that shared, when it comes down to you, I don't need to tell you that most weight-loss plans don't work over the long term. You inherently know this. That's why I understand if you're feeling cautiously optimistic about Protein Pacing. You're probably hopeful that this will be the routine that changes your body—and your life—for good. You're also probably not quite ready to give away your baggiest pair of pants, but your mind is getting set right at least! I get it.

Believe me when I assure you that this program is different. Remember my nickname, "Dr. Metabolism"? If you read through part 1, you have learned that for better or worse, I really am this single-minded. My greatest passion (after my family and maybe tennis) is finding ways to help people feel great while losing fat, gaining muscle, improving health, and fitness. Through my work, I've helped tens of thousands of people release massive amounts of body fat, especially harmful belly fat, all while maintaining or increasing lean muscle mass through my laboratory research studies, private coaching, and research breakthroughs.

Now millions have heard about my programs through my speeches and media appearances.

From the get-go, my primary research goal has been about improving health through changing a person's body composition, reducing fat, and increasing muscle tone so they're performing at peak condition. I just knew that there was a way to get the body to burn more fuel by optimizing what, when, and how a person eats and what type of exercise they did. It took a few decades (and dozens of extensive scientific studies beginning back in 1988) to hone in on the ideal formulation, but several years ago I finally devised the perfect nutrition plan, one that I wrote up for the March 2013 edition of the highly regarded scientific journal *Obesity* and have since reproduced in several ground-breaking, landmark published studies.

In the first-of-its-kind study, I detailed how men and women who followed a reasonable, deprivation-free Protein Pacing diet plan, without any exercise, were able to shed pounds—up to 5.5 pounds in one week and 11 pounds in four weeks. This weight wasn't just water loss. "I calculated fat loss too, and some dieters shed 12.5 pounds of body fat, including 2.5 pounds of belly fat, all while building lean body (muscle) mass (up to 4 pounds!) after just eight weeks! That means belts tightened, dress sizes dropped, and body changes could be felt and seen. In a recent follow-up study, I tested my Protein Pacing plan in a group of forty overweight men and women and in twelve weeks they lost an average of 10% body weight or 24 pounds, with some losing up to 65 pounds, 9 inches off their waist circumference, and 46 pounds of fat! Including more than 4 pounds of belly fat!

Remarkably, despite the massive loss of body weight and body fat, the relative amount of healthy lean muscle mass increased by 9%! In seven follow-up studies I added exercise to the Protein Pacing equation (using my PRISE protocol details I am sharing with you in the next part) and the results were off the charts—by adding four short workouts a week to this program, you could lose as much as 22 pounds in four weeks! And these results are not just for those interested in weight loss. I've tested my PRISE Protocol on super-fit men and women, and they out-performed their non-PRISE counterparts in every measure of physical performance too! This is why this is not a diet, it is not a temporary fix, it is a lifestyle plan that will work the rest of your life. Imagine, finally knowing that you can end the diet roller coaster and settle in for the rest of your life in an excellent, not too intense, great tasting, satiating, never hungry, "non-diet," eating for life program and one that keeps you healthy and does not deprive you.

The Protein Pacing Plan

The "rules" of the Protein Pacing eating plan came from all these years of performing my own research and from reading scientific studies from my colleagues at institutions like Duke, The Mayo and Cleveland Clinics, Columbia, Penn State, McMaster University, and Cornell universities. To create a weight-loss program that offers both short-term and long-term success, I pulled the best parts from each of these plans, meshed them together with some of my own work, and landed on an eating routine that leads to the best results I've ever encountered. Still to this day!

So just what is this magical lifestyle formula? Well, it's not nearly as complicated as you might think. In fact, it borrows from principles that you may have seen before. Here are the basics of the Protein Pacing plan:

1. ◊ Each Protein Pacing snack or meal should include high-quality complete protein of all twenty amino acids from either animal or plant-based or a combination of both.
2. ◊ Each snack or meal should contain 20–40 g of high-quality protein
3. ◊ Eat a minimum of four and a maximum of six Protein Pacing snacks or meals.
4. ◊ Evenly spaced (about every three to four hours) throughout the day.
5. ◊ Eat your first Protein Pacing meal sixty minutes from waking in the morning. This is what I refer to as the Morning Muscle Maximizer (MMM).
6. ◊ Eat your last meal within two hours of going to sleep at night. This is what I call Bedtime Bellyfat Burner (BBB).

When it comes to eating, quality and moderation—not deprivation—are key to controlling cravings and sticking with a healthy lifestyle for good. If you want to lose weight, place the right amount and type of protein (20–40 g) and fats (saturated, monounsaturated) on your plate and less starchy carbohydrates.

Here are some other things I've learned to complement Protein Pacing; four to six meals a day keeps your metabolism roaring and decreases your chance of unplanned snacking, as long as you are eating protein at each of these meals! Eating the right carbohydrates keeps your blood sugar and insulin at healthy levels. Fueling your body with the right fat can help decrease inflammation in your blood vessels, enhance brain and nerve function, and provide an excellent energy source for physical activity. Natural whole and nutrient-dense engineered foods—not heavily engineered nutrient-deficient ones—are best because they contain the ideal amount and ratio of cancer-fighting phytonutrients, vitamins, and minerals necessary to help us prevent disease and perform at our best. By eating foods that are more filling, you won't miss any extra calories you give up.

You'll learn more about what exactly I recommend you eat and avoid later in this book. For now, just know that when I tested hundreds of people on the PRISE Protocol they experienced weight loss so significant I was sure they were hungry or deprived or were tired, which are common side effects of consuming too little fuel. *They weren't!* Instead, these men and women lost fat, flab, jiggle, and belly rolls, all while feeling better than ever. And you can too! The Protein Pacing plan is designed to help you burn more fat calories all day long and build more lean muscle all the while keeping you feeling satisfied and not hungry. Many report experiencing a happier, less-stressed mood state as well on the Protein Pacing meal plan.

The beauty of Protein Pacing is that it can fit into anyone's busy lifestyle and food preferences, intolerances, and allergies. Below, I show you how easy it is to include my Protein Pacing plan into any nutrition/diet plan you choose. For example, the growing popularity of the plant-based, Mediterranean, paleolithic, and fat-adapted/ketogenic diets meet the needs of those of you wanting to "kick start" your weight loss or enjoy an athletic performance advantage over your competition. By using my *original* Protein Pacing plan with proven scientific results, you'll follow a diet of roughly:

30% protein
30% fat
40% carbs

Whereas, if you want to follow the:
Protein Pacing *plant-based* plan, you will consume:

20%–25% protein
15%–20% fats
60%–70% carbs

Protein Pacing *fat-adapted/ketogenic* plan, you will consume:

20% protein
70%–75% fat
10%–15% carbs

Protein Pacing *Mediterranean* plan, you will consume:

20%–25% protein
25%–30% fat
50% carbs

Protein Pacing *paleolithic* plan, you will consume:

20%–30% protein
50%–60% fat
20%–40% carbs

Regardless of which type of overall nutrition plan you choose, Protein Pacing is always the "foundational core" of each one of them! (I provide examples in appendix A) This is why I'm am so passionate about spreading the word on Protein Pacing. It is the common nutrition thread to EVERY nutrition/diet plan available!

My *original* Protein Pacing plan is the basic formula followed by all the men and women in my research studies, including the *Obesity* study who lost weight, and how you will too. The average American diet already consists of 50% carbs, 16% protein, and 34% fat[63], so we're only talking about small changes to what you eat, not a full diet overhaul. That should make this program a lot less

---

63   Centers for Disease Control and Prevention. June 02, 2009. Accessed February 18, 2018. https://www.cdc.gov/nchs/data/hus/hus16.pdf#056.

daunting than some of the others out there—you're already on the right track. By cutting back on things like soda, candy, and starchy carbs and adding healthy protein from grass-fed, free-range, wild, organic animal sources (including whey protein), and organic, local, plant-based sources, as well as healthy fats to your meals, you'll get the scale to start moving in the right direction.

SAMPLE Protein Pacing MEAL PLAN

MEAL	FOODS
Morning Muscle Maximizer (Breakfast) 20–40 g of Protein	**Choice of:** Shakes, Smoothies, Pancakes, Waffles, Muffins, or Bowls with fresh fruits and veggies: Multi-vitamin with adaptogens & antioxidants
Mid-morning Snack (Optional) 20–40 g of Protein	**Choice of:** Bowls with grains, nuts, seeds, fruit, veggies, dark chocolate; Bars, Shakes, or Smoothies: Optional; Natural-sourced caffeine beverage with antioxidants & adaptogens
Lunch 20–40 g of Protein	**Choice of:** Shakes or Smoothies; Fish, Poultry, Beef, or Pork (grass-fed, wild, free-range); Legumes and Grains (quinoa, millet, amaranth, brown/wild rice, etc.). All with fresh veggies and fruits
Mid-afternoon Snack (Optional) 20–40 g of Protein	**Choice of:** Bowls with grains, nuts, seeds, fruit, veggies, dark chocolate; Bars, Shakes, or Smoothies: Optional; Natural-sourced caffeine beverage with antioxidants & adaptogens
Dinner 20–40 g of Protein	**Choice of:** Fish, Poultry, Beef, Pork (grass-fed, wild, free-range); Legumes and Grains (quinoa, millet, amaranth, brown/wild rice). All with fresh veggies and fruits

Bedtime Bellyfat Burner (Evening Snack) 20–40 g of Protein	**Choice of:** Shakes, Bars, Smoothies or Puddings with fresh or powdered veggies, fruits, and nuts/seeds. Add Dr. Paul's Sleeping Aids of magnesium, calcium, vitamin D, tart cherry juice, pumpkin seeds, melatonin, valerian root, and air-mist of lavender oil

*Drink plain water and with electrolytes throughout the day. Shakes/Bars/ Smoothies/Pancakes/Waffles include either animal and/or plant- based protein sources (whole foods and powders) such as; un-denatured whey, egg, pea, fava, mung, brown rice, pumpkin, collagen, etc. Bowls include probiotics and may be either animal and/or plant based sources from dairy, almonds, cashew, flax, pea, quinoa, oats, cassava root, tapioca, chia, locust bean, hemp, coconut.

For some people, combining my Protein Pacing with any of the diet plans I list above may result in even more dramatic improvement in body composition. This is what makes my Protein Pacing plan so effective; it can be adapted to any healthy diet plan and boost your results to the next level. I share this with all of you who may be interested in an exploration of your human potential. By incorporating my Protein Pacing plan with your nutrition/diet plan of choice (such as a plant-based, Mediterranean, paleo, fat-adapted/ketogenic diet), you may find that you have greater energy, a decreased desire for unhealthy food, improved mood, and greatly improved body composition. Combined with the metabolic increase, greater satiety, and improved protein synthesis you will gain from the Protein Pacing plan, you can take your lifestyle to the next level of performance.

After I created the *original* plan, I became interested in the recent trends in *fat-adapted* or *ketogenic* eating strategies. So, what does it mean to be "fat adapted?" As it turns out, human beings have been around for quite a long time, much longer than cookies, cake, breads, soda, and all of the other high-carbohydrate, refined, and starchy foods that many of us love so much. How did human beings survive for thousands of years without pasta and all of its starchy compadres? It's coming to light that a large majority of the human diet was historically made up of protein, animal and plant fats, along with whatever fruits and vegetables were in season and naturally occurring. How diets have evolved when humans were first hunter-gatherers is what has given the paleo diet traction today. A ketogenic or fat-adapted diet may seem extreme, and indeed it is night and day in comparison to the foods that many of us choose to eat on a daily basis, but a diet with the right types and amounts of fats can help you to unlock the full energy potential of all of your stored fat! Imagine: you have the potential to feel consistently satiated while also getting rid of all of your unnecessary body fat at the same time!

With a fat-adapted diet, you can train your metabolism to use fat as the primary energy source. This means that even while at rest and exercising at moderate intensity, you will be primarily burning fat as fuel. Recent scientific research on "thinking evolutionary" when it comes to dieting has even demonstrated that high-fat diets have the potential to turn on aspects of the human genome, stored within us, that help us to burn and utilize greater proportions of fat in our diets, the way our ancestors did. A fat-adapted diet is comprised of generally 60%–70% fat, sourced from healthy saturated and monounsaturated fats. The rest of your dietary needs are satisfied by healthy proteins (healthy and well-cared-for animals have the benefit of also containing delicious and healthy fats as well) using my Protein Pacing plan (~20%) and minimal carbs. The carbs that you do eat will comprise 10%–15% of your dietary intake and will be largely resistant starch and nutrient-dense vegetables and greens.

The difference and speed at which body fat is released may be truly exceptional. And, in case you have concerns that this is dramatically different or too complex routine, just take a peek (appendix A) at some of the minor differences to help you understand it better.

While it is exciting to see the extra effect the fat-adapted ketogenic diet offers, it still remains controversial for many experts so proceed with caution. Regardless, you have to follow those basics about the use of my Protein Pacing plan whether you choose the fat-adapted, plant-based, Mediterranean, Atkins, or paleolithic diet. To be clear, Protein Pacing is *NOT* a high-protein diet. As I stated earlier, it's the right type and amount of protein at the right time. And don't be fooled by all those "posers" who claim we are eating too much protein; in fact, just the opposite is true. Remember that well-respected and validated scientific data I shared? As the worldwide obesity epidemic has ballooned since the 1980s, data shows we are eating too many carbohydrates, especially simple sugars, during this same time period, and protein intake has decreased!

Thus, Protein Pacing holds the key to healthy weight loss and optimal performance. Several human nutrition intervention studies from my research laboratories provide strong support for following my Protein Pacing plan to decrease total body weight and body fat (including abdominal and harmful visceral fat), increase proportion of lean muscle mass, and improve cardiovascular and metabolic health. Our study diets range between 20–40 g per meal of high-quality animal and plant-based protein that emphasize foods such as nuts/seeds, legumes, beans, pea/brown rice protein powder, free-range eggs and poultry, grass-fed dairy products (milk, Greek yogurt, cottage cheese, whey protein powder), wild fish, and grass-fed beef.

Of course it would be amazing to eat these healthy and tasty protein foods throughout the day. But, the reality is, many of us simply do not have the time, energy, or money to prepare and purchase these foods for every meal we eat; this would be a full-time job!

Instead, I recommend we combine high-quality whole foods and nutrient-dense engineered protein powders and bars to maximize the Protein Pacing plan effects, and I have the science to back it up. For example, sound science has proven that four to six meals per day containing 20–40 g of protein per meal from both protein-rich foods and powders and bars (such as naturally sourced unde-natured whey and plant-based protein shakes and bars) stimulates metabolism up to eight times more than fat and two and a half times more than carbs; opti-mizes protein synthesis needed for enhanced repair and building of lean mus-cle mass; and quenches hunger better than any other nutrient. All of this helps maintain an ideal body composition leading to optimal health and peak perfor-mance. Here is a chart that shares some ideas of what protein to use. An easy way to keep track of your Protein Pacing plan each time you eat a meal or snack is to use the palm of your hand as the serving size for any animal-based product, such as beef, chicken, turkey, fish, eggs; the size of your fist for a plant-based protein serving, for example, quinoa, chick peas, tofu, legumes, and lentils; and one to two scoops of undenatured whey or plant-based powders in the form of brown rice, bean (fava, mung, etc) and pea protein.

Protein Pacing Meal/Snack Options (20 g servings)

Key points to remember: 1) consume at each of your four to six daily mini-meals beginning with breakfast; 2) adjust from 20 to 40 g as needed; 3) consume immediately after exercise; 4) consume a serving two hours prior to going to bed

Quick Reference Guide:

Legumes (choose dry version):

Black beans, chickpeas: 8oz (1 cup)

Kidney beans: 13.5oz

Lentils: 8oz (1 cup)

Nuts & seeds (unsalted, dry-roasted):

Peanuts, dry roasted, unsalted: 3.5oz

Peanut butter: 5 tablespoons

Almonds, dry roasted, unsalted: 3.5oz

Cashews, dry roasted, unsalted: 4.5oz

Sunflower seeds: 3.5oz

Pumpkin seeds: 4.0oz

Flaxseed, ground: 3.5oz

Wheat germ: 2.75oz

Fish:

Salmon: 3.5oz

Tilapia: 3oz

Haddock, halibut: 3.0oz

Cod: 3.0oz

Swordfish: 3.0oz

Tuna/mackerel/sardines in can: 3.0oz

Egg:

Cooked egg white: 4 eggs

Hardboiled, scrambled eggs: 3 eggs

Egg substitute: 7oz

Protein Powders & Supplements:

Undenatured whey protein concentrate, isolate or hydrolysate: powders (1 scoop of 20–30 g), in meal replacement bars (range from 15–30 g per bar). Brown rice, fava, mung, legume, or pea protein (1–2 scoops of 20 g). Bone broth or collagen protein powder or liquid.

Yogurt:

Greek yogurt, plain (non-fat): 8oz (1 cup)

Greek yogurt, plain (2%): 8.5 oz (1 cup)

Kefir, plain (low-fat): 14oz Yogurt, non/low-fat, plain: 16oz (2 cups)

Cottage Cheese:

Non-fat cottage cheese: 5.5oz

1% Low-fat cottage cheese: 6oz

2% Cottage cheese: 8oz

4% Cottage cheese: 7oz

Milk (organic):

Skim: 21oz (2.5 cups)

1%, plain, chocolate: 20 oz (2.5 cups)

Meat (choose local, free-range, grass-fed, whenever possible):

Lean beef, sirloin, buffalo: 3.5oz (avg of all cuts)

Chicken breast, w/o skin: 2.5oz	Turkey breast, w/o skin: 2.5oz
Chicken, dark meat, w/o skin: 2.5oz	Turkey dark meat, w/o skin: 2.5oz
Sliced turkey or ham: 3.5oz	Pork chop: 3oz
99% fat free ground turkey: 3oz	Pork tenderloin: 3oz

To break things up and clear your head from the facts for a moment, I'm going to tell a personal story. It is about how life has changed through the years, but it is something that you can keep in mind because we all seem to be on the run these days. My first introduction to what I now call a road warrior (RW) occurred during my childhood watching my dad, a traveling clothes salesman, prepare for the work week every Sunday. His routine involved organizing and packing huge bags of clothing samples he would carry up from the basement, one by one, and load into the trunk of his car.

It was an exhausting way to start the work week, and it didn't stop there. Every day during the week he would go through the same routine along his "territory route," unloading and loading each clothing sample bag at each of the department stores and private retail shops he visited. At the time, I didn't pay much attention to the physical demands of his job as a traveling salesman. But now, I fully appreciate and marvel at what he accomplished each week for more than thirty-three years!

Without question, it was his diet (okay, and bag lifting) that kept him healthy, strong, and mentally prepared throughout his career as a true RW. Similarly, many hard-working men and women continue to hit the pavement, train tracks, or airways as RWs, and a healthy, nourishing diet is crucial to keeping them on top of their A game when they reach their destination. We often have to treat our lives the same way.

I hate to say it, but one of the largest barriers to being successful in a lifestyle routine is consistency, even while we are on the run or living our hectic lives. We need to think and plan ahead and figure out ways to always have nourishment at our fingertips while we are rushing, or in the office, in places that are not conducive to healthy eating, at parties, and the list goes on. But once we get into the habit, it will become second nature to be prepared. I hope this little story makes you relate and want to be with the best of the RWs—prepared and ready to take on a healthy life!

To help you, here are some strategies I put together to provide the necessary foundation:

Protein Pacing for All of the Road Warriors:

Rule #1: **Eat 20–40 g of protein at each of your meals,** especially important at your "power lunches" to keep you mentally sharp and energized. Too often, poor food choices at lunch turn "power lunches" into "weakness lunches," and we feel sluggish and energy depleted.

This protein stabilizes blood sugar, replenishes energy stores, nourishes muscles and brain, and revs metabolism.

Plan to eat 0.7–0.85 g of protein per pound of body weight per day. Most packaging on food contains this information.

For example:

150-pound person should eat 105–128 g of protein per day (150 x 0.7 = 105 g; 150 x 0.85 = 128 g)

*If you add exercise to your daily routine, add an additional 20–25 g immediately following your exercise session. Individuals above sixty years old should aim for the higher level of protein intake (0.85 g per pound of body weight).

Rule #2: **Eat a protein- and fiber-rich breakfast**. Starting the day with a 20–40 g serving of protein and 8–10 g of fiber revs your metabolism, quenches hunger, and promotes healthy lean body mass (muscles). Other added benefits are increased mental focus and you stay "regular."

Rule #3: **Pack a cooler**. Stuff the cooler with water, cut veggies, fresh fruit, Greek yogurt, cottage cheese, homemade protein smoothies, natural peanut butter with rice cakes, homemade hummus, trail mix, hard-boiled eggs, protein bars, and your favorite stuffed pita or sandwich wraps. If nothing else, it keeps hunger pangs in check and drastically reduces the likelihood of binging on fast food.

If you plan to be driving all day, restock the cooler at a grocery store along the way. This also provides an opportunity to get out of the car, stretch, walk around, and pick food you want, instead of sitting at a restaurant or, worse yet, a fast-food drive-up window and order only what is available on the menu. I highly recommend grocery store pit stops en route to your destination.

It's more difficult to restock at a grocery store when traveling by train, so plan ahead and pack some extra protein bars. Your goal is to feel nourished, energized, and thinking clearly when you arrive at your destination.

Rule #4: **Eat Protein Pacing every three hours** with last serving within two hours of going to bed at night. I recommend traveling with a protein bar (providing ~20–30 g of protein) or protein powder (24–36 g) to mix with water whenever hunger strikes.

Air travel is the most time-efficient method and allows us to arrive at our destination the quickest, but it's also the trickiest environment to maintain a healthy eating plan. Restrictions on size of carry-ons make bringing food a challenge. This is unfortunate because air travel food (airports and planes) often suffers in taste and quality.

Regardless, packing food for air travel is the same—higher protein, nutrient dense, and convenience. Excellent choices are protein bars, powders, and home-made trail mix. During flight, choose fresh veggies and fruit, yogurt, and trail mix, and always opt for water or tea to drink.

Finally, before I conclude this chapter, I want to add two other timing, pacing, and success strategies that you definitely want to try to get into your daily routine as soon as possible. One is what I call the Morning Muscle Maximizer (MMM) and the other the Bedtime Bellyfat Burner (BBB)! These are two more daily commitments that will assure that you get the right type of protein into your body at the right time.

Thirty years of metabolism research has taught me: 1) starting your day with a nourishing protein-rich breakfast provides significant health benefit, 2) maintaining Protein Pacing meals evenly spaced throughout the day will optimize body weight control and enhance body composition, among many other health and fitness benefits, and 3) ending your day with the right type of protein at night will keep your metabolism working even while you sleep!

Despite these truisms, there are still too many non-believers. My published research[64], as well as research by others, supports my Protein Pacing nutrition method beginning first thing in the morning at breakfast (MMM), this is the "bulls-eye" that cannot be missed. Unfortunately, there is too much noise and misinformation in the media and even among certain scientists and health experts that take a limited and often incorrect perspective of current dietary intake trends, and this includes the obesity epidemic data from the US Department of Agriculture from 1950–2000, as well as numerous research studies that compare one high-carbohydrate breakfast to another. In reality, recent peer-reviewed scientific data paints a much different picture of food intake trends, prevalence of obesity among Americans from 1970–2010[65], and beginning your day with a protein-rich breakfast. While both sets of data agree that food intake increased approximately 200 calories per day during this time period, the source of where those additional calories come from differs drastically.

The problem is there continues to be enormous media attention and controversy surrounding the topic of whether breakfast is an important meal of the day. This topic is especially popular at the beginning of the school year when parents, teachers, administrators, coaches, and children are scrambling to prepare for the start of school. Unfortunately, the truth of whether breakfast is an important start to a productive day is often missed or neglected. Despite a flurry of recent news articles suggesting that breakfast eaters are not healthier than breakfast skippers[66] the "science" says they are.[67] As a definition of "healthier,"

---

64   Arciero et al. Studies listed in Bibliography; specifically 2008; 2013; 2014; 2017. *Am J Clin Nutr*: 2011,93:836-43; 2013;97:848–53.

65   Ibid.

66   Additional media attention:

   Peter Whoriskey, "The science of skipping breakfast: How government nutritionists may have gotten it wrong." *The Washington Post*. August 10, 2015. Accessed March 18, 2018. https://www.washingtonpost.com/news/wonk/wp/2015/08/10/the-science-of-skipping-breakfast-how-government-nutritionists-may-have-gotten-it-wrong/?utm_term=.60d3aca497fa.

   John Berardi, PhD, "Breakfast: Not Really the Most Important Meal of the Day." *The Huffington Post*. December 15, 2013. Accessed March 18, 2018. https://www.huffingtonpost.com/john-berardi-phd/breakfast-health_b_4436439.html.

   "Is breakfast really the most important meal? Why a new study says maybe not." TODAY.com. Accessed March 18, 2018. https://www.today.com/health/new-study-says-breakfast-may-not-be-most-important-meal-t37991.

67   J. I. Baum, M. Gray, and A. Binns. "Breakfasts Higher in Protein Increase Postprandial Energy Expenditure, Increase Fat Oxidation, and Reduce Hunger in Overweight Children from 8 to 12 Years of Age." *The Journal of Nutrition*. October 2015. Accessed January 22, 2018. https://www.ncbi.nlm.nih.gov/pubmed/26269241.

   H. J. Leidy, H. A. Hoertel, S. M. Douglas, K. A. Higgins, and R. S. Shafer. "A high-protein breakfast prevents body fat gain, through reductions in daily intake and hunger, in "Breakfast skipping" we mean improved body weight control and body composition management and in some cases better brain power and mental performance.

I'm here to help you understand why there appears to be confusion over the question "are breakfast eaters healthier?" First, most of the published research on the topic of breakfast and health has compared only two conditions: 1) skipping breakfast or 2) eating a high-carbohydrate sugar-sweetened breakfast cereal and juice. As you would expect, the skipping breakfast condition often resulted in more favorable health outcomes because starting your day with a stomach and body full of sugar is not good. Thus, the news reports summarized that eating breakfast is overrated and less healthy than skipping it altogether.

Fortunately, more well-controlled recent studies have incorporated a third condition—eating a high-quality protein breakfast—to allow for a comparison of the "quality" of the composition of the breakfast meal. The overwhelming conclusion of these recent studies clearly shows that a high-quality protein breakfast is indeed healthier than skipping or indulging in a typical high-carbohydrate breakfast. While most of the studies have focused on weight control and body composition, a limited, but growing body of research is measuring cognitive and academic performance as well. A summary of the findings from these studies also supports a reduced consumption of simple carbohydrates for improved cognitive performance.[68]

Therefore, the "take-away message" is start your day with a nourishing protein- and fiber-rich breakfast (containing 20–40 g of high-quality protein and 5–10 g of fiber) to provide significant health and performance benefits. I refer to this as the *Morning Muscle Maximizer* (MMM), and it's part of my Protein Pacing meal plan that has as its first strategy "to eat your first Protein Pacing meal within an hour of waking in the morning. The number one reason for this is because your body is in a state of protein breakdown by the time you wake in the morning following an overnight fast, and this is not an ideal environment to preserve and build healthy lean muscle mass. Thus, starting your day with a Protein Pacing meal to initiate protein synthesis to help maintain and start to

adolescents." *Obesity* (Silver Spring, Md.). September 2015. Accessed March 18, 2018. https://www.ncbi.nlm.nih.gov/pubmed/26239831.

68   Valeria, Rosato, Valentina, Maria, Gabriella, Lorenzo, Emilio, Monica, Decarli, and Adriano. "Effect of breakfast composition and energy contribution on cognitive and academic performance: a systematic review | *The American Journal of Clinical Nutrition* | Oxford Academic." OUP Academic. May 27, 2014. Accessed March 8, 2018. https://academic.oup.com/ajcn/article/100/2/626/4576549.

build healthy lean muscle mass is your top priority and makes the MMM one of the most important meals of the day, without question!

Protein holds the key to weight loss, especially if it's consumed first thing in the morning for breakfast as part of my MMM. Several recent intervention studies from our laboratory provide strong support for eating a Protein Pacing diet, especially at breakfast—to decrease total body weight and body fat (including abdominal/visceral fat) while improving heart and metabolic health.

And for the evening? Incorporate my Bedtime Bellyfat Burner or BBB. I've warned you about the dangers of excess body fat. I've even taught you about the different types of stored fat. Let me dive in just a little deeper. The most abundant site for fat storage is just beneath the surface of our skin, called subcutaneous fat. Subcutaneous fat is found all over the body and has a tendency to accumulate in larger amounts centrally around the abdomen (belly) in men and is referred to as android fat and given the name "apple shape." In women, subcutaneous fat deposits accumulate in greater amounts around the hips and thighs and is called gynoid fat or "pear shape." When excess fat accumulates in the belly (android) region, some gets stored deeper and surrounds the vital organs, such as the heart, liver, kidney, and pancreas and interferes with the normal healthy functioning of these organs. This deeper storage of fat around the vital organs is termed visceral fat and leads to significant disease risk for diabetes and heart disease, including high blood pressure, obesity-related disease, and even certain cancers. [69] We want to do everything in our power to get rid of this dangerous visceral fat, "belly fat." As I describe above, men are more likely to store excess fat in the belly and, therefore, have greater visceral fat and disease risk. However, women of post-menopausal age are at similar risk for visceral fat accumulation and thus disease risk due to changes in hormones (lack of estrogen).

Unfortunately, given our current nutrition and food landscape around the world, more and more people are at risk of excess abdominal belly fat and visceral fat disease risk, including young boys and girls. The main reason for this disturbing public health concern is likely due to excess calorie intake, especially refined simple sugars. In fact, recent research has shown a link between higher simple sugar intake (sugar sweetened drinks) and higher visceral fat levels in

---

69   Heval Mohamed Kelli et al., "Changes in Body Fat Distribution Is Associated with Oxidative Stress," *Journal of the American College of Cardiology* 69, no. 11 (2017): doi: 10.1016/ s0735-1097(17)35184-7.

adolescents (fourteen to eighteen years old).[70] Perhaps most alarming was the finding in those with the highest sugar drink intake also showed the highest levels of the stress hormone cortisol upon waking in the morning. Talk about an addictive response! We are creating a toxic environment for our children by making available to them an overabundance of sugar-sweetened drinks, which may be altering their stress hormone levels by the time they awake in the morning, all of which is associated with a significantly greater accumulation of the dangerous visceral fat. Something has to change.

This something is exactly why I've developed the PRISE Protocol and especially Protein Pacing. My research and others has consistently shown that the timing of when you eat protein near bedtime may have a beneficial impact on our visceral fat. My research over the past ten years has consistently proven that when a bedtime Protein Pacing snack is provided within two hours of going to bed at night—as part of my overall Protein Pacing plan and what I refer to as the BBB—with and without exercise training, visceral fat always drops drastically.[71] This is exactly why I want you to start to incorporate this tonight. Don't delay!

You can have a protein smoothie using 20–40 g of undenatured whey protein or a combination of pea, legume, seeds, and brown rice protein powder mixed with 6–8 oz. of tart cherry juice, magnesium powder (250 mg), and a handful of pumpkin seeds. Or if you'd rather chew on something, have a high-quality protein bar containing 20–35 g of whey protein concentrate and isolate or pea, legume, seed, or brown rice protein for a great night's sleep and continued belly busting results even while you sleep! [72] Again, you can use any of the healthy protein sources I mentioned in the above chart; just make sure you start MMM and BBB today. That's not a lot to ask.

I hope you now agree that the science of eating a breakfast with protein and a protein snack at bedtime are truly Protein Pacing answers. You really can start

70   G. E. Shearrer et al., "Associations among sugar sweetened beverage intake, visceral fat, and cortisol awakening response in minority youth," *Physiology & Behavior* 167 (2016): doi: 10.1016/j.physbeh.2016.09.020.

71   Paul Arciero et al., "Protein-Pacing Caloric-Restriction Enhances Body Composition Similarly in Obese Men and Women during Weight Loss and Sustains Efficacy during Long-Term Weight Maintenance," Nutrients 8, no. 8 (2016): doi:10.3390/nu8080476.

72   G.E. Shearrer et al., "Associations among sugar sweetened beverage intake, visceral fat, and cortisol awakening response in minority youth," Physiology & Behavior 167 (2016): doi: 10.1016/j.physbeh.2016.09.020.

to get rid of the visceral fat and start to feel better. You may wake up in the morning feeling more refreshed than you have in years. I want you to follow the valuable strategies in this chapter as a road warrior, pacing the times during the day that you eat protein, but never forgetting to use them for breakfast and bedtime. You will feel great and be on top of your game! Throughout the centuries, we were more protein-based eaters. But hunter-gatherers of the old days didn't eat an 18-oz. steak every meal of the day. Our early ancestors ate what they hunted and often consumed foods that were high in fat to sustain them through times of famine. We then supported our quick energy needs with fresh fruits and vegetables. This is what made us strong enough to go out and tend to the land or hunt for our meat or pick those fruits and vegetables from the wild. Mother Nature has taught, and continues to teach, us everything we need to know. We simply need to start listening.

I understand that in today's fast-paced world, we all seem to lack that most essential element called patience, but with a little preplanning, with the process and all the steps in order for you as I have done—even when it comes down to types of protein and when—you can take the frustration out of the process and each little gain (meaning loss of pounds!) is going to prove worth the wait. Isn't it time you adopted the evolutionary pace of nature and never diet again?

With following the protein concepts alone, I hope I have created a new sense of purpose for you in the journey you are about to take. Remember, as you keep your eyes on the prize using the power of protein and the key of pacing, and even though my research subjects lost weight with just this, imagine what happened when they added exercise to their routines? Of course, that is the topic I will focus on in part 3.

> *"The best time to plant a tree is twenty years ago. The second best time is today."*
> — Stephen M.R. Covey, *The SPEED of Trust: The One Thing that Changes Everything*

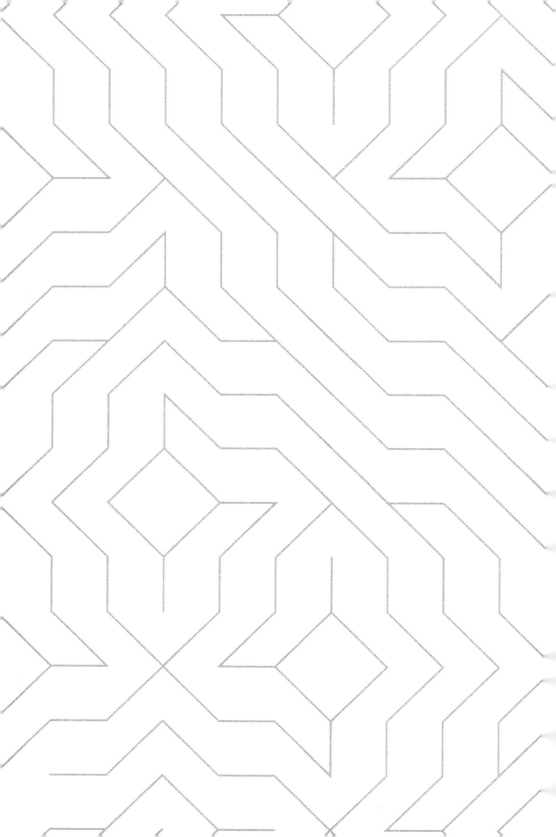

PART THREE

Dr. Paul's PRISE Life Protocol Revealed

Simplicity is the ultimate sophistication.
—Leonardo Da Vinci

Time to RISE Up! (Fitness Is . . . LIFE . . .)

P—PROTEIN PACING

R—RESISTANCE

I—INTERVAL

S—STRETCHING

E—ENDURANCE

9

The Story Behind the PRISE

"Never get so busy making a living that you forget to make a life."
—Aristotle

Who knew my early start with the PRISE Life actually began when I was competing as an athlete eager for new ways to enhance my performance and recovery from training and competitions? It exploded when others started looking to me for advice, but the next journey I am going to share ends with a *very different moral* to the story than you may guess, so please read to the very end.

In my peak athletic competition years, I launched myself into reading all sorts of nutrition, physiology, and scientific-based research to help me improve. But, over time, more and more people started asking me what I was doing to stay in shape and perform at a high level. The *sharing* of this information with others actually became *more* fulfilling and motivating to me. As I shared at the beginning of the book, the major "spark" that ignited my passion to pursue a career in helping others achieve optimal health and peak performance was in response to watching loved ones, including my grandparents and father, suffer from disease. It started my career as a nutrition and exercise scientist. But when I knew I "arrived" was when my research was being accepted in peer-reviewed publications, in leading science journals, and I was sought as an invited speaker at various national and international nutrition and sports medicine conferences. I was quickly becoming one of the go-to content experts. The top athletes wanted to know what I was doing and soon, so, too, was the regular person looking to get healthy and fit. As a matter of fact, as word got out around town, when I would send out announcements in local newspapers for interested study participants to learn more about enrolling in one of my upcoming research studies, I was blown away with the number of people who would show up in my small community just for the information meetings—sometimes as many as 240 people! This is unheard of in terms of human clinical intervention studies that involve a nutrition and exercise program. I knew I was on to something special and word spread very fast.

In the past, I've been asked on radio shows and in media how to summarize why or how I came up with this protocol. I was also asked to share this in my book. It might surprise you, but I *would* say I developed PRISE because current exercise and nutrition recommendations are too time consuming, confusing, and not realistic for the majority of people. And that is *part* of the truth. That is why less than 20% of the United States population achieves them on a regular basis, whereas, in the research studies I have done on PRISE, my adherence/compliance is often 80% or higher! Compare that to the national average of less than 20% of people who meet the current exercise guidelines. That's astronomical! People report loving PRISE because it's easy to follow, fun, has variety, time efficient, social, can be customized or individualized, flexible, and consistently produces results. People report their excitement because they don't feel like they are being held hostage to a diet and exercise plan but feel as though they can actually incorporate this as a lifestyle change for the rest of their lives. Now, that's proof right there of its success!

I do talk about a lot of the steps that led up to my discoveries in my presentations, but essentially, I came up with PRISE in response to our current exercise and nutrition recommendations from the leading organizations in the world including American College of Sports Medicine (ACSM), American Heart Association (AHA), The Obesity Society (TOS), and Institute of Medicine (IOM). Current exercise recommendations are very well-intentioned and well-meaning; however, they are much too aggressive, confusing, and not feasible for the vast majority of the population to achieve. Hence, why less than 20% of the United States' population meets the current exercise guideline recommendations and perhaps even less with nutrition guidelines.

Interestingly, and to make sure we are moving in the right direction, I have been a Fellow in the ACSM since 1997, I served on the AHA advisory board, and I'm a Fellow in the TOS and the International Society of Sports Nutrition (ISSN)—all prominent and leading players in the global health, fitness, nutrition, and wellness space. Most importantly, my research is cited in the current

ACSM exercise recommendations *position stand* as well as the leading sports nutrition organization in the world (International Society of Sports Nutrition). This means I truly am the respected and heeded scientist contributing to the current exercise and nutrition recommendations.

In a sense, I took very complex material and varying philosophies on exercise physiology and nutrition and brought it back to the basics of what was actually being recommended. I performed a simple calculation on the number of hours necessary to accomplish the current recommendations, and it requires up to nine to fourteen hours a week or one and a half hours per day of exercise! Few people have that kind of time to exercise every day of the week because, as I said, it holds you hostage and is much too overwhelming for most people. Not only are the current recommendations too extreme and time consuming, but they are also confusing to follow and, most importantly, make no connection to healthy eating. Thus, I wanted to develop a more sensible, realistic, time-efficient exercise routine that embraced all of the important components of the current exercise requirements but were also seamlessly connected to a healthy nourishing nutrition lifestyle strategy. This was how PRISE was born. Or, as I said at the start of this chapter, so I thought.

The very strange thing about life is that we often don't know what is motivating us while we are "deep in it," and it's not until we are forced to slow down or asked to summarize our lives that all of a sudden we get new perspectives. In chapter 1, I spoke about feeling like I was looking down at the earth and could finally see the cross sections... well, *poof,* all of a sudden two days ago, I had an epiphany. And just to share, please realize I was almost done writing this book, when wham it hit me! Then, as I sat down to write about it, I couldn't believe my eyes when someone shared this quote by Aristotle: "Never get so busy making a living that you forget to make a life." The timing was perfect because I had just gone through this *massive* revelation about my own personal life, had literally just shared it with my wife the day before, and this quote appears! Has that ever happened to you? It's amazing how timing can be perfect and how little hidden signs pop up along the way to show we are on the right track.

Anyway, what happened is that I had been forced, or all right, strongly encouraged, because of writing this book, to think further about how I pioneered Protein Pacing along with the PRISE Protocol, and all of a sudden, it was like the blinder's had been taken off of me. I always thought it was because I was looking for the best way as an athlete to reach peak performance, to be on top, and that is still largely true, but it finally hit me that it was much more than that. The fact is, I created this protocol out of *survival*. When I look back now at this journey, I can't even believe I made it through to share this! I think you will agree and even empathize.

I say *survival* because that is the absolute truth as to what it was. Early on my professorial and scientist career when my wife, Karen, and I had two young sons (we are blessed with three now), they were ages one and three at the time, we both had full-time jobs, and were juggling trying to have a marriage, have new roles as parents, deal with regular life stress, balance new careers, pay the bills, and juggle all of life's pressures. I call it the "Struggle of the Juggle". All of that with one huge monster on our backs: our impossible schedules with absolutely no downtime. After you read this, you will realize that we must have been crazy, because who in their right mind would have kept this up? And, spoiler alert, we did it for twelve years at max velocity! My wife and I still question each other on what took us so long to wake up and realize how much we sacrificed along the way and needed to think through this and get out of the rat race, or at least off the wheel! It's probably because we were functioning in *survival* mode and never took a breath to contemplate what we were really doing and what the consequences were. I'm sharing this because there is a very real possibility in today's world that you are in exactly the same spot we were.

Let me give you just a little background so you know there was a method to our madness, at least in my mind at the time. After graduating with my two masters, my doctorate, and postdoctoral fellowship training, I was fortunate enough to get a full-time faculty position at a prestigious four-year liberal arts college as an untenured professor and head men's tennis coach. Let me explain. Back in those days, there were only a few colleges that allowed professors to teach academic courses and also coach an athletic team. And, the few who did, were primarily in a field that was called Physical Education or Kinesiology. If they did any research they were either doing it through the humanities or education departments of most colleges. I, however, accepted this job to be a college professor and scientific scholar with a lab. With that position I was also given the position of Head Tennis Coach. That's right, I was the two-for-the-price-of-one guy. Yup, my total salary of $32,000 a year, untenured faculty, (for a family of four) came with two jobs—and may I say, two jobs that had completely opposing schedules, while Karen was working as a physical therapist and an amazing mom to two beautiful new babies.

In my job as a scientist, I even took the harder route. Did I choose to work with cells? No. Animals? No. Microbes? No. I chose to work with human subjects! Yup! Leave it to me. Other scientists joke that they have more flexibility because when working with a rat or a cell you can do it on your time, or at least control the time. Working with a human, not just a human on their time, but on the time of human metabolism, meant that starting at 5–6:00 a.m. on every laboratory testing day, I had to be in the lab taking samples and working with my subjects. (If you're a farmer, you might be saying, "That's nothing. I'm up every morning seven days a week milking the cows!") Well, I agree, but that was just the start to my day. I was up really early, leaving my wife to care for the babies. I would run into the lab, get my tests done, run home when that was done to help feed the babies breakfast, then scoop them up so my wife could get to work (physical therapist). I would drop the boys off at daycare, which, thankfully, was the building next to mine, work through the day, teach classes, grade papers, do research, prepare for my classes, grade exams, serve on committees, write manuscripts for publication, apply for grant and research funding, etc. And by about 4–5:00 p.m. when the college was clearing out and going home to be with their families and rest up, where was I headed? Well, to my job as Head Tennis Coach, of course! It started at about 4:00 p.m. when the athletes would show up and practice, and work would begin. This could go up until 7:00 p.m. or later in the "off" season. But if there are two "off" seasons, there are two "on" seasons and, yes, that was fall and spring when we had championships and other tournaments.

What did that mean? It meant that we had extra practices and at all the oddest hours because we had to book court space. So, as if getting up to be to work at 5:00 a.m. was not enough, I rushed to the lab, got the kids to daycare, and there was the added 6:00 a.m.–8:00 a.m. extra practice court time on weekends or, just as grueling, the 10:00 p.m. to midnight practices during the work week. I am telling you, looking back now, our life was nothing short of *brutal*. Yes, you read it correctly. There were days that I started before 5:00 a.m. and got off after midnight. But that's not all. Did the college have its own van and a designated driver for my tennis team? Nope. Then, there were the weekend tennis matches. As coach, on a Friday night when all were going home by 5:00 p.m., my wife was dropping off cookies and cakes with two kids on her arms so that I could drive my team the three to six hours to the location of the competition. If it was Maine, there was a five-hour ride! Think about this: I was gone all Friday night, all Saturday, and late into Sunday eve, never able to be with my family and only to get home to grade papers, plan my lessons, do my research, write up information, keep the committees happy, and I was *even* in charge of recruiting. If your head is spinning in circles, to be honest, the more my wife and I discussed this, the more we couldn't believe we did it for so long—twelve years! Don't get me wrong, the main reason we stayed doing this so long was because my wife and I considered my players and students our adopted children; we loved them and would do anything for them. But life was stressful for sure.

Can you imagine spending so little time with your children and young wife and spending all these hours working around the clock? I had no assistant at work; I had no extra help. *Brutal.* Now, imagine running that much on so little. What does that do to a person? Well, because I was a scientist and health, nutrition, and fitness was my field, I knew I had to keep up and remain emotionally balanced and fit. But how? With absolutely not a spare moment in my life, how was I supposed to exercise and even eat right? Without knowing it, and in survival mode, what did I do? I *created* my own plan! Yes, one that was effective and healthy and didn't take as much time as my profession told me it should. Now do you see what I just figured out? I created a nutrition and exercise plan for people who have *no* time. Can you believe I only realized this portion a few days ago?

I started focusing on the fact that time was of the essence, and I needed to incorporate the healthiest and quickest eating and staying healthy program I could find. I was not going to sacrifice my love for my family. I had to figure out how to get some exercise in, how I could maintain my muscle strength and function, and perform my job at work and as a devoted husband and father without getting fatigued. I couldn't risk letting anyone down or letting my job duties slip because I was too tired, ill, or hurt. I had to figure out how to properly stretch in limited times, and I had to figure out how to keep my heart functioning at peak levels to build endurance because I was literally on the run for my life! This was the most absurd, chaotic, and crazy life I could imagine, and I was trying everything in my power to stay alive and healthy while achieving my goals and maintaining my responsibilities for career and family. Throughout all of this, my number one priority was staying close to my family, and when this was challenged, I went into "high alert" mode. It is often reported that the greatest contributions, inventions, and achievements are "born" out of survival and protection of loved ones. In my case, PRISE was due to both.

All this leads me to *you*. I needed to find balance. I was somehow creating it despite the chaos and lack of minutes in the day. I was doing what almost every person today does, and most of us, honestly, find overwhelming. I was trying to balance relationships with family and career. I was trying to keep up financially to care for my family, pay bills, pay for daycare, make sure my human research studies were treated with the utmost care, teach my students, coach my athletes, and stay at the top of my game for $32K a year. I had to learn how to remain nourished and be able to exercise to the point of optimal health when I had no time to commit! Sound familiar?

I made the commitment and that is what I did, a full twelve years, until the day the college came to me and gave me a choice. Ironically, they, not me, realized that my two full-time jobs were pretty close to humanly impossible. Therefore, they came to me, and I was given the choice to either be a professor/scholar-scientist or Head Tennis Coach. And as you can guess, I chose professor/scholar-scientist.

I am grateful to the administration for realizing that what I was doing was impossible and perhaps, because they were looking from the outside in, they could see those circles I was running in that I couldn't see myself. And, please, don't misunderstand me for a minute; I loved my jobs, my school, and my students, but why couldn't I see what I was doing to myself and my family when I was so deeply entrenched? It is a question that a lot of us ask after the fact, but I am asking you now. Are you doing the same thing? Are you running in circles or finding it so hard to keep up that you can't see what or why you are doing it? Is there a better way? Can that way start now?

I feel blessed to have been able to get all this experience so quickly, but a funny story happened after the college approached me and I had chosen the scientist over coach job. When they hired that new head coach on full salary, and rightly so, you know the annual salary I had gotten for *two* jobs? The person came in, and guess what? Along with the salary, they even gave him an assistant! You read that right! An assistant. I never had an assistant. Remember, I was that new father who was spending weekends away from his family to literally drive the team to tournaments on top of working two jobs. I'm not blaming the college; those were different times. But as I said, when my wife and I started really looking at the past, we realized that time and how much we endured.

This is where we now go back to the fact that we were too caught up to see anything. We were spinning in circles as fast as we could just to keep up. We didn't have time to think about what we were doing. We had little balance for the most part, and I can assure you, like all married couples, when it came to the "big" fights, just like you, they were centered on finances and not spending enough time with the family. And who could blame Karen or me for being overwhelmed and taking it out on each other? The good news is that we made it through these times much stronger as a couple and a family, and we continue to find more and more balance yearly. But the point is, I don't want you to live through what we did. I want you to learn from our mistakes and that means, first, stop, take a breath, and ask yourself, "Is everything I'm doing really necessary?"

I want you to ask yourself that question seriously. Why? Because one of the largest research groups I ended up studying included working moms juggling life, career, kids, family, money, health, finances, love, stress, and the list goes on. I would look at their commitment (and the busy men as well) and realize that so many of the people who strive to do well, watch what they eat, and try to get in exercise are the same overachievers that I am guilty of being. I want you to think about that now, because you have now become my target group. The group that I want to help slow down and balance. The ones I want to help reassess what they are doing in their multitasking days and teach how to take the nutrition and fitness portion to an easier and permanently doable level so that they don't one day move so fast they fly off that wheel and end up "broken" because they forgot to pay attention!

Ask yourself now, "What can I let slide to get quality back into my life, and who can help me?" The beauty of my life's lesson may not have been balance back then, but out of this was birthed my eating and exercising protocol that will help put balance back into your life. I want you to embrace my program because the good news is that, with millions as living proof, you can achieve optimal health and peak performance even with a limited schedule and living on the run.

The moral to this story: If we had a chance to do things over, I would *never have gotten so busy making a living that I lost, forever, the time to make a life*. Fortunately, I was learning as I was going through it all, and as my PRISE Protocol became more and more refined, I was able to spend more and more time with Karen and my kids. They were, and always will remain, my PRISE. Please, please do not make the same mistakes I did. Together we are all going to hold each other accountable to work smarter and *not* harder! You promise? I do. I'm committed to making life better for all of us.

Now that you have even more of an understanding that my entire goal in creating this program is for those who are on the run and lacking time, I'll bet I have your attention. My "survival" has become your prize—because as they say, necessity is the mother of all invention, and I assure you trying to stay healthy with that insane schedule was a necessity!

Amazingly, through these three decades, one of the most astonishing results of my research still stands: What we are being taught and told to do in the area of nutrition and exercise has missed the target and may actually be causing more harm to our bodies versus healing and strengthening us. Every time I share my work and see results, I feel more driven to share this with the world. I have made this protocol relatively simple and definitely easy to follow, and that is one of the reasons it is so successful for the time-deprived.

I'm excited to show you how to incorporate each of these lifestyle strategies into easy-to-follow steps as part of your daily life, so you can reach optimal health and peak performance. It is easier than you might think! This is for the moms who don't have a minute to think, to say nothing about blink, the fathers and family members who are caring for sick loved ones while working full-time jobs, while going to school, while paying the bills, while trying to put good food on the table, all while constantly on the run. This is for you!

And, as I say, I don't want to just sit in the ivory tower from the science lab; I'm taking it to the streets! I want to get this to everyone to stop obesity, poor health, and help the world learn that you don't have to fall for the misinformation out there. Have the courage to put your belief in this. You really can and will achieve success by following the systems I present. Failure is no longer an option. You will find that this protocol is the answer to Aristotle's sage advice: "Never get so busy making a living that you forget to make a life."

10

R-RESISTANCE
Lose the Fat: Gain the Muscle!

Resistance
I
S
E

It is finally time to tackle the topic that scares most people off or brings great dread to anyone other than an athlete—and even the tired and frustrated athlete who doesn't want to train at times. The word is *exercise*. This is why I will do my best to use the word *fitness* instead. Fitness has a much more positive meaning to people, because it's what we all aspire to achieve in our lives. The great news is that it no longer needs to be a burden. First, because you see how this lifestyle program has success even without fitness (a little reverse psychology tip). Second, because you have control over your fitness and choosing what you like to do; therefore, it can actually become fun!

In the studies I performed, you noticed that I did not make fitness a requirement to make sure that we could gather true statistics. But for real life, fitness is necessary and good for you. The good news is you don't have to do as much as you have been led to believe or work as strenuously as you may have been told. Everything I teach will help you build lean muscle and get rid of the harmful belly fat, especially that dangerous visceral fat.

I know that anyone starting a new fitness program wants all the hard work and sweat to pay off in some way. Some of the more common payoffs include body weight and fat loss, toned muscles, increased energy, better mood, and improved athletic performance.

However, statistics tell us that most people who begin a fitness program don't receive these payoffs. Why is this? Many current fitness programs are to blame for this high failure rate because they are too intense and time consuming and hold us hostage by expecting us to work out like a "fitness-aholic" nearly every day of the week! None of us should be pushing ourselves to the brink of physical exhaustion every day thinking that this is the *only* way to achieve fitness, health, and wellness. While you may experience a few positive results in the short term, it does little, if anything at all, to keep you motivated in the long term.

Recently, I came across this statistic. More than 60% of Americans (or two out of three people) make New Year's resolutions, mostly to get healthier (>85%), but only 8% are successful in achieving their resolutions.[73] Why is this? How can so many well-intentioned and determined people fail at such a noble, worthwhile, and healthy cause? We have an abundance of easily accessible information on how to get fit, eat healthy, and manage our stress, so it's not a result of not knowing what or how to do it. Or is it?

In my own experience working with tens of thousands of people on a regular basis from all ages, fitness levels, and health statuses, the most common complaint I hear on their quest to become healthier is "I don't know what to do or how to do it!" In other words, despite the massive amount of fitness information we have at our fingertips, most of us struggle making sense of it or having a clear understanding of what steps to take. It has become a case of "(mis)-information overload" that has created confusion, frustration, and an epidemic of inaction, leading to the opposite effect of what it was designed to prevent—poor eating habits, physical inactivity, stress, and disease.

I have devoted my life's work to helping others navigate the nutrition, fitness, and wellness landscape in an easy-to-follow path leading to optimal health and peak performance. Before I introduce each of the PRISE fitness components, it's important to follow four important steps: 1) obtain clearance from your health-care professional to begin participating in a fitness program, and nearly all of them will be thrilled to support you on this mission; 2) learn how to choose an appropriate exercise *intensity* to avoid injury and benefit from the

---

73   Dan Diamond, "Just 8% of People Achieve Their New Year's Resolutions. Here's How They Do It." *Forbes.* January 02, 2013. Accessed January 14, 2018. https://www.forbes.com/sites/dandiamond/2013/01/01/just-8-of-people-achieve-their-new-years-resolutions-heres-how-they-did-it/2/.

exercise; 3) choose appropriate dynamic warm-up and cool-down exercises; and 4) don't forget to have fun. To make this second step easier for people, I have developed Dr. Paul's PRISE Intensity Scale for Fitness (see appendix B) to help you perform the fitness routines at a level that is safe and effective for improving health and performance. To make the third step easier, I have developed recommended exercises with explanations (see some examples in appendix C, but I do have an exercise journal and handbook if you want the full routine). By following these routines, it will be easier for you to create a core program that becomes second nature versus reinventing the wheel.

The most common mistake people make when they begin a fitness program is exercising at the wrong intensity level. For example, some exercise too vigorously and get injured and don't enjoy it, while others don't push hard enough and don't see any results. In both cases, the end result is most of them quit!

If you're going to take the time to exercise, you want to get the biggest payoff possible. That means finding the intensity that is best for you, whether it's finding the right amount of weight to lift or the perfect speed to walk or run. If you don't push yourself enough, you won't make the gains you want. You will build muscle and zap calories, but not as quickly as you could. If you go too hard, you risk injuring yourself, sidelining yourself for a few workouts to several weeks. Of course, how much you should do depends on the type of exercise you're trying and the intensity you work at.

Dr. Paul's PRISE Intensity Scale for Fitness (appendix B) is an effective solution to help people choose the proper exercise intensity so they reduce their risk for injury, see results, and enjoy it! My scale will serve as a helpful guide when performing the RISE fitness routines. I encourage you to use the scale on your own for the next month, but aim for a level of 4–6. Then, as you progress, you can slowly work to increase intensity level at a safe pace.

Another important factor as you consider the intensity level is to make sure you warm-up and cool down. This is way more important than you realize. Many exercisers treat the warm-up and cool-down portion of a workout the same or, worse yet, skip them entirely. But both are essential. A proper warm-up heats your body so it's ready to move the way you want it to. A proper cool-down stretches out some of the muscles you just challenged, making you ready for your next session. A warm-up should be active, including walking and movements such as leg and arm swings and circles. A cool-down can be active and static, including a cool-down walk and stretches such as toe touches. Aim to add five to ten minutes of warming and cooling activity at the front and back end of all of your workouts. I always recommend that before starting each **PRISE** exercise routine, perform a walk/jog warm-up for five minutes at a moderate pace (Intensity Level 4–5). I have included a complete listing of Dynamic Warm-up exercises in my exercise journal and handbook, but some samples are included in appendix C to help you with ideas and to show you form.

I want to share another little segment of hints and suggestions for those of you who may not have made fitness a habit and are trying to get back into it. There are some basic guidelines that will help you decide to become fit, especially if you are on the fence or find you just need one little excuse ("Oh, gee I forgot my lucky workout shirt in the dryer!") to bow out, with the key being prepared at all times. These steps may seem simple, but you would be surprised how using them will get you in the mood to succeed.

Dr. Paul's PRISE Protocol Fitness Tips to Success

Before you start PRISE, please download the PRISE App so you can take it with you anywhere, anytime to guarantee success!

1) **Prepare ahead to avoid any excuse.** Some people keep spare clothes in the car or put them on the way out the door, so they don't have to search for a swimsuit or exercise shoes or a towel or a yoga mat—it is right where you can see it, not only to remind you, but to help you lose the excuses as to why you can't exercise today.

2) **Schedule your workouts.** In order to get the benefits of fitness, you actually have to do it. If you're like most people I know, fitness is the first thing to fall off when your schedule gets full. By actually blocking it out in your calendar, this is less likely to happen. You can also recruit a workout buddy to keep you on track. When your alarm rings at 6:00 a.m., you may want to hit snooze. But if you know your friend is waiting for you at the park or gym, you'll be a lot more likely to get up and going.

3) **Fuel and hydrate right.** What you eat and drink throughout the day will either sabotage or boost your response to fitness. Remember…

what you eat *exceeds* any amount of fitness you do *all* the time. The goal is to have food/drink intake and fitness work in synergy, not against one another. Within one hour of starting your fitness routine, plan to drink 8–16 oz. of water. (This will help you stay hydrated, even if you sweat a lot.) Also, be sure you eat something within two or three hours of starting. A small meal (think 200–300 kcals) of fresh vegetables or fruit, lean protein, and whole grains can help you stay strong from start to finish. If you're exercising less than an hour, water is all you usually need to drink. If you are exercising for more than an hour (or in hot and humid environment), have a sports drink containing glucose (sugar) and electrolytes (sodium, potassium, chloride, magnesium, calcium, etc.) on hand to keep you workout-ready. Sip as you exercise to stay energized and hydrated.

4) **Dress the part.** Wearing the wrong shoes or clothing for a workout can make you uncomfortable and set you up for injury. Choose comfortable and appropriate fitting clothing and footwear for each type of exercise. If you're worried your sneakers may be worn out, buy new ones so you get the support you need. It may sound silly, but I always recommend fitness newbies do a dress rehearsal for their workouts to make sure their gym bags have all the right gear and their workout outfits fit right and provide the right blend of stretch and support. Nothing shuts down good exercise intentions faster than socks that bunch up when you walk or shoes that rub the wrong way. The type (mode) of fitness will determine the appropriate clothing and footwear needed. For example, the fitness session may require a bathing suit, cycling or running clothes, yoga or weight training clothes, layered clothing for outdoors, and a change of clothes. Be prepared for changing conditions, and bring a stopwatch to stay on time. What you wear does make a difference.

The Acronym PRISE

As you can see, PRISE is an acronym, the "P" for Protein Pacing and the "RISE" exercise portion, which I will define below. The entire PRISE Protocol is synergistic and works perfectly when you implement the four exercise components together. It trains your muscles, lungs, heart, and mind, turning your body into an even more efficient fuel-burning machine. The workouts are all under an hour long, and you only have to fit in each workout once a week. That means that less than four hours of exercise a week can help you double—or triple!—your weight-loss results.

To accelerate your results and firm as you burn, you'll combine Protein Pacing with my signature exercise series, RISE, which helped dieters in my studies lose more weight more quickly. It preserved their lean muscle mass as well as enhanced performance outcomes among already super-fit women and men. The best part of PRISE is that it's individually tailored to your own personal health and fitness goals to ensure you achieve maximal results in the quickest time possible. Because it's so easily customized to each person, it's not uncommon for an eighty-three-year-old woman to perform a PRISE exercise routine alongside a twenty-four-year-old world-class athlete! That is an exercise program with longevity!

PRISE is revolutionizing how the scientific and medical community prescribes and recommends exercise to the entire population and is the "change agent" we've all been looking for to finally make an impact on the epidemic of obesity and lifestyle-related diseases but also to create the next wave of world-class athletes.

RISE stands for:

◊ Resistance exercise—Resistance training includes traditional strength training, of course, but also includes more functional resistance exercises that use only your body weight or the addition of rubber bands, tubes, physioballs, medicine balls, and other mobile strength training devices. It involves contracting your muscles against a force and is the best method to increase muscular function, strength, power, and build endurance.

◊ Interval exercise—Interval training includes specific types of short bouts of quick and intense movement of your larger muscles with recovery periods in between. It is the best form of fitness training to develop a lean, sculpted body composition of increased lean muscle mass and decreased fat mass (total and abdominal), as well as heart health and metabolic health and fitness.

◊ **S**tretching—Stretching training involves all types of stretches and poses (yoga, tai chi, qigong, etc.) that enhance blood flow and is the most effective fitness training to increase your muscle/tendon flexibility, joint mobility, and create a deeper mind–body connection.

◊ **E**ndurance—Endurance training includes all the different exercises that keep your heart and muscles pumping for long periods of time in a full-body rhythmical manner to produce the greatest cardiovascular health benefits and feelings of euphoria, happiness, and mental function (executive function, decision-making, etc.).

I will show you how to perform each of these different but highly beneficial fitness training routines to give you the greatest opportunity to achieve optimal health and peak performance in the most time-efficient manner possible. There is no arguing the scientific proof I've established supporting my PRISE Protocol to produce amazing results in people of all ages, health, and fitness status.

Here's a sample PRISE Protocol for a week:

Sunday	Monday	Tuesday	Wednesday	Thursday	Friday	Saturday
Protein Pacing						
REST	RESISTANCE	RECOVERY	INTERVAL	STRETCHING	RECOVERY	ENDURANCE

Note: PRISE **R**ESISTANCE exercises utilized medicine balls, physioballs, rubber tubes, and bands, which were incorporated into dynamic warm-up, footwork and agility drills, resistance and power movements, core exercises, and bodyweight exercises (e.g., lunges, squats, and jumping rope). **I**NTERVAL AND **E**NDURANCE exercise modalities available include: walking, jogging, running, cycling, swimming, elliptical, rowing, rollerblading, cross-country skiing, etc.

Another schedule I've recommended that also includes intermittent fasting looks something like this:

Monday = Resistance
Tuesday = Recovery
Wednesday = Intervals
Thursday = Stretching
Friday = Recovery
Saturday = Endurance
Sunday = Recovery (intermittent fasting)

Resistance
I
S
E

Resistance: In the PRISE Protocol, the resistance routines are focused on developing muscular strength, power, and even endurance. So, your workouts will focus on building lean muscle mass by using a combination of traditional weights (dumbbells, barbells, fitness equipment) but focus primarily on your body's own weight as resistance, plus the use of small props such as an exercise band/tube, medicine ball, or kettlebell. You'll work the large muscles first, overloading them, before focusing on your smaller muscles. This type of resistance training zaps total body and belly fat, increases lean muscle mass, and improves cardiovascular and metabolic health as well as enhances your mood. The muscle mass you could gain from this type of exercise is impressive. In my PRISE study, some participants packed on close to 8 pounds of lean body mass in twelve weeks! That's over a half pound of muscle a week—the type of strength gain you can quickly see and feel. One women I worked with went from being able to do just nine push-ups to mastering over twenty-five at a time; another was able to bench press an extra 25 pounds. All this from less than two months of working out! Women, don't worry; you won't walk out looking like the Incredible Hulk, but it will define your muscles, especially your upper body, and that visceral fat (bad fat on your belly) and hip fat will start to disappear! When you perform the resistance training routine, aim to keep your intensity level between 7 and10.

RISE with Resistance

There are hundreds of ways to get in your resistance training, or strength training. You could use the leg press machine at your gym, do biceps curls with the use of a resistance band at your house, or even hold a plank position in your office. You can use weights or props to provide resistance and challenge your muscles, or you can stick to moves that use your own body weight, such as squats, lunges, pull-ups, or push-ups. In other words, there's no excuse not to integrate resistance workouts into your routine.

Of course, I do have my own preferred methods for building lean muscle. PRISE is built on the premise of working the large muscles first. This type of training allows you to gain the most benefit, because you overload your muscles from strongest and largest to weakest and smallest. My scientific research and experience with clients and athletes shows this type of training reduces total body and belly fat, increases lean muscle mass, and improves cardiovascular, metabolic, and mood health. By building more muscle, as you do when you work the larger muscles like the glutes and quadriceps, you burn more calories, lose body fat, lower blood pressure, and increase your overall strength. Even if you're mostly interested in building strength and creating a more toned physique, you'll automatically get these other benefits too.

Resistance Training 101

I've given a few examples of resistance moves—things like biceps curls and squats—but here's a more in-depth explanation of how it works: Resistance exercise includes any physical movement that requires muscles to exert a force against some sort of resistance, whether it's gravity or a dumbbell. This force against resistance causes the muscle cells, sometimes referred to as fibers, to contract and change length.

Most resistance exercises result in shortening of muscle cells. These are concentric muscle contractions, such as a bicep curl. However, some resistance exercises cause muscle cells to lengthen. These are known as eccentric muscle contractions and include movements such as lowering a heavy weight to the floor. Lastly, a major component of my resistance training is a form of muscle contraction called plyometrics. These are exercises that require the muscles to be rapidly stretched ("loaded") and then immediately contracted, such as jumping off of a box onto the ground and then jumping onto another box (box jumping) or performing push-ups with a clap between them. The goal of plyometrics is to improve muscle power. Whichever way the muscles are working (shortening or lengthening), they respond favorably to resistance training by improving the blood supply and nerve conduction pathways to our muscles. It's sort of like construction work on a highway that adds another lane to make room for more vehicles and allows for easier transportation. The result is a more efficient transportation system to increase the speed in which oxygen and nutrients are delivered to help muscles repair damage and rebuild new muscle. Just as important, chronic resistance exercise training may also help remove waste and release toxins that build up in muscles. The enhanced nerve pathways lead to smoother and faster-firing muscles, which is a very good thing. Taken together, the improved blood and nerve supply results in leaner muscles and better functioning and performing muscles.

The bones and joints also respond favorably to resistance exercise. Most people feel healthier, stronger, more fit, and better able to accomplish tasks and activities of daily living like climbing stairs or lifting heavy objects when they resistance train. You may find that your bone density scans improve when you start lifting weights and that your joints actually feel less achy thanks to the extra support your muscles are providing. I'm never surprised when I hear a test subject with arthritis in her knees say she's feeling a lot better after regularly doing lunges and squats.

For athletes, the increase in muscle function results in improved explosive power, strength, and agility, which translates to improved athletic performance. Runners and cyclists who add strength training to their routines are able to move faster for longer periods of time. Sports players may be able to jump higher or throw harder. Strengthening your muscles may allow you to lift heavier weights, but it'll also allow you to move better in all the things you do.

The following is a chart that I created to make the process easy to follow:

PRISE: Resistance (R) Exercise Routine

Circle the Exercises Performed from Each Category		Reps/ Time	Intensity
Dynamic Warm-up (Appendix C)	**Perform prior to each workout (Choose 7; 1 set; 7 minutes):** 1. Pendulum swings (side to side) 2. Pendulum swings (front to back) 3. High knee (chest) 4. High knee (external rotation) 5. Side shuffle 6. Carioca 7. Over-under the fence 8. Hip opening/closing 9. High knees 10. Butt kicks 11. Lunge with twist 12. Arm windmills		
Footwork & Agility	**Perform using agility ladder (Choose 4; 1 set; 4 minutes):** 1. Forward, double-step 2. Sideways double-step 3. Side-step, double in/out 4. Side shuffle, two-in/out 5. Two leg hops 6. One leg hops 7. Two leg hops, in/out 8. One leg hops, in/out 9. One leg hops, sideways 10. Side shuffle 11. Figure 8s 12. Kangaroo hops 2/1 foot 13. Kangaroo hops, sideways 14. T-drill 15. Jump rope		
Resistance & Power Exercises	**Perform 6 below (2 sets; 12 minutes):** 1. Side-steps toes in/out, ankles/knees - Side-steps with bands and med ball 2. Forward/backward walk with bands 3. Squats		

Resistance & Power Exercises cont.	4. Lunges with tubing (with med ball)
	5. Lateral lunges (with med ball)
	6. Front step-ups
	7. Squat thrusts, med ball throws
	8. Jump squats
	9. Mountain climbers
	10. Squat-plank-jump squats
	11. Lateral step-ups
	
	Perform 6 below (2 sets; 12 minutes):
	1. Back rows/fly
	2. Pull-ups
	3. Chest press/fly
	4. Pushups (**choose one**):
	  - side walking
	  - knees/toes w/physioball
	  - down dog
	  - side to side (ball)
	  - heart-to-heart
	  - hi/low
	5. Front/Lateral raises
	6. Biceps curls
	7. Shoulder press
	8. Hyperextensions		

Core Exercises	**Perform 5 below (2 sets; 10 minutes):** 1. Plank knees elbows/hands 2. Plank toes elbows/hands 3. Plank one leg elbows 4. Plank one leg hands on ball 5. Side planks foot-elbow/twist 6. Side planks hand stars 7. Airplanes 8. Superwoman/mans 9. Crunches on ball 10. Plank with ball on knees/toes **Perform 5 below (1 set; 5 minutes):** 1. Knees to chest 2. Hyperextension on ball 3. Reverse planks 1,2 legs 4. Ab hollow		

Core Exercises cont.	5. Walking sit-ups 6. Crunch bent knee 7. Tug-of-war 8. Side touch/scissors/toe		

*Cool down five minutes following R routine with gentle stretching. Total R exercise time is ~50–60 minutes.

Building on Your PRISE Resistance Training Plan

PRISE contains an expansive and continuously growing number of resistance training options, and I've included many of them above, but they are also included in my PRISE App (Apple App Store and Android Play Store). Remember, the resistance exercise training program is a series of exercises that incorporate dynamic, functional resistance movements of footwork/agility drills; body weight exercises involving weighted medicine balls, physioballs, and exercise tubes and bands; along with core strengthening exercises. Perform each exercise with enough weight or intensity (Intensity Level 7–10 using my scale) that your muscles are fatigued after either 30–40 seconds or 10 to 20 repetitions per set. You can change how hard you're working by lifting a heavier weight, using a thicker resistance band or tube, a heavier medicine ball, or moving more slowly or quickly.

Resistance exercises are absolutely wonderful and essential to getting stronger, healthier, and increasing your physical performance. The beauty is they don't have to be limiting. Don't forget that exercise can be done in places other than just the gym. Consider bringing along my PRISE travel gym to the park, office, vacation, or business trip. I designed it so you can perform these routines anywhere, anytime. One thing to keep in mind is doing anything is usually better than nothing when it comes to general physical activity. Some little tips I recommend: park at the furthest destination from your office, store or event; leave your lunch in the car until you arrive at your office and then walk back out and get it; every hour walk to a co-worker in another building or on a different floor; when reading, watching TV or performing deskwork at home and work make a point to stand up for 10-15 minutes every hour and stretch; carry shopping/grocery bags versus using a cart; practice diaphragmatic breathing (belly breathing) whenever you're feeling stressed; and when waiting in line or at the airport do some simple stretches. Any moment you have a chance to cherish nature, get outside or *just* breathe. And never, ever forget to have some fun! Bop in the pool, add a little tango to your warm-up, jive to some music, rap to some pumps, and by all means, remember that exercise was meant to be enjoyed, not torture! Don't take yourself too seriously in the beginning by comparing yourself to the perfect ones in the gym. You are there for you, and soon you will be so thrilled you may be helping others!

Use your mind to pretend you are Andre Agassi, one of the Williams sisters, Gretsky, an Olympian, whatever gets your mind to help you move is not only allowed but *encouraged*. Your body, in its perfection, will have those endorphins pumping in no time, and you will finally start to enjoy it, "RISE Up," and actually want more of this exercise thing! No more excuses! So, when you are smiling to yourself in the gym or accidently grunting Serena or Nadal style, smile at yourself with pride or turn to your partner and say, "Dr. Paul told me to RISE Up!" That will be our little secret. But how you lost the fat and gained that muscle is something you can shout out to the world, especially as people start to ask you what you are doing to look so good. And remember, I'm constantly conducting new research studies on the effects of my PRISE Protocol using the best nutritional support available to maximize your results. So, visit my websites often to stay on top (www.paularciero.com, www.proteinpacing.com and www.priseprotocol.com).

Websites

11

I-INTERVAL Sprint through Life: Relish the Afterburn

R
Interval
S
E

Drive slow and enjoy the scenery—drive fast and join the scenery.
—Douglas Horton

"Slow and steady wins the race" is an often repeated saying that reminds us to slow down and take our time. This, of course, comes from the famous Aesop's fable of the tortoise and hare in which the overconfident, speedy rabbit challenges the turtle to a race and, despite sprinting away from the turtle at the start line, ends up falling asleep during the race and eventually losing to the slow-moving turtle. As a result, one take-away message is that it doesn't pay to "sprint" through life.

However, when it comes to your health and fitness, "sprinting" in the form of high-intensity sprint **Interval** exercise is one of the most effective and efficient types of exercise to burn fat, build muscle, strengthen the heart, and increase metabolism. Research shows that staggering slow and fast segments of cardio is one of the best ways to improve your health. To do an interval, you're going to walk, jog, swim, row, or cycle super fast, then slow enough to recover and catch your breath. This sort of exercise improves cardiovascular fitness, increases lean muscle mass and metabolism, and reduces body fat, belly fat, and blood sugar. Plus, it's quick! With intervals you can exercise for less than thirty minutes, yet you'll be stronger and feel more energized when you finish. This is a good way to gain fitness fast. With intervals, some of my PRISE testers improved their cardiovascular fitness by more than 80% in eight weeks. That means no more huffing and puffing up the stairs!

When it comes to your health and fitness, sprinting during high-intensity **Interval** exercise is one of the most effective and efficient types of exercise to help you reach your fitness and weight goals. What do I mean when I say "intervals?" Interval training is often shown using a ratio of exercise to rest or work to recovery. For example, you might do one minute of work then recover for two minutes. It's these changes in intensity that make a workout an interval workout. You work hard and fast, and when you're about to tucker out you take a short break—usually to catch your breath—then you do it all again.

And please don't be fooled into thinking that intervals are only for the top elite athletes. Research consistently shows that intervals are one of the most effective and safest training strategies for the obese, type 2 diabetics, and cardiac rehabilitation patients![74] In other words, intervals are great for everyone, no matter your fitness or health status or age or gender. So let's start sprinting together. The people I work with love intervals because they are so time-efficient—exercise for less than thirty minutes and you'll feel stronger and more energized when you finish. Interval training can be applied to just about any type of aerobic activity, including walking, jogging, swimming, or cycling. If you can speed it up or slow it down, you can add intervals.

Interval Training 101

Most people think the best way to lose body fat, especially belly fat, is through endurance or aerobic exercise; the opposite is actually true. A growing body of scientific evidence shows that interval training is the best way to enhance aerobic fitness and turn your body into a fat-burning machine! Not

74 Some specific studies that prove my points:
O. Rognmo et al., "Cardiovascular Risk of High- Versus Moderate-Intensity Aerobic Exercise in Coronary Heart Disease Patients," *Circulation* 126, no. 12 (2012): doi:10.1161/circulationaha.112.123117.
Kassia S. Weston, Ulrik Wisløff, and Jeff S. Coombes, "High-intensity interval training in patients with lifestyle-induced cardiometabolic disease: a systematic review and meta-analysis," *British Journal of Sports Medicine* 48, no. 16 (2013): doi:10.1136/bjsports-2013-092576.
Romeo B. Batacan et al., "Effects of high-intensity interval training on cardiometabolic health: a systematic review and meta-analysis of intervention studies," *British Journal of Sports Medicine* 51, no. 6 (2016): doi:10.1136/bjsports-2015-095841.

only do intervals add excitement to your usual cardio routines, but they are a much more time-efficient way to fitness and leanness. So, instead of heading out for a steady run or bike ride, carefully monitor your time, going hard or easing up based on how you feel using my intensity scale and by what your watch says in terms of the time or heart rate. Your brain will be busy, and your body will be working in a new and challenging way. But this isn't some simple diversion tactic. Intervals really do make your workout effective. Research shows that staggering slow and fast segments of cardio is one of the best ways to improve cardiovascular fitness; increase lean muscle mass and metabolism; and reduce body fat, belly fat, and blood sugar.

Interval training automatically improves fitness. Most people are aware that when you run at a steady state, such as when you set the treadmill to 6 mph, your body gets into a rhythm. This is perfect for *endurance* training—if you tap out at thirty minutes one day, you might be able to eke out thirty-two minutes the next, and so on. Your body gets a little bit stronger with each workout. What most don't realize is that this is true for intervals. You can increase your endurance in the same way, but you'll also be increasing your power and speed.

For example, say you're that person who regularly runs at 6 mph. What would happen if you were to bump up your speed to 8 or even 8.5 or 9 mph? You could probably keep up for a short period of time, such as thirty to sixty seconds. After that, you'd have to come back down to a very slow walk of 2.5 to 3 mph to catch your breath. That's how intervals work. You step outside of your comfort zone, building muscular endurance as well as speed and power. Over time, if you practice this way you'll be able to sprint faster and faster. It might take you less time to get to your top speed, and you will be able to sprint faster and faster as time goes on. I tend to recommend that people start training with a 1:3 interval ratio—one minute of all-out exercise for every three minutes of recovery. As your fitness levels improve, you might notice that you need a slightly longer time to recover because you are pushing yourself even harder during the sprint interval.

Part of what fuels this gain in speed, endurance, and power is a gain in muscle tone. When you really push yourself, you're bound to grow muscle fibers. As you already know, this increase in muscle leads to a boost in daily calorie burn. For each pound you add, you can expect to burn around an extra hundred calories a day. However, that's just one way intervals lead to a higher all-day calorie burn.

One of my favorite aspects of intervals—and one you're going to love too—is a change in several key enzymes inside our muscle cells that create the "afterburn."

In science speak, afterburn means the period of time you continue to burn extra energy (or calories) after a workout. Although you may be done exercising, your body is still in a high metabolic state, which means you're zapping extra calories automatically. Imagine that you sit for an hour and, in doing so, burn sixty calories. (As you know, sitting is not the answer for weight loss!) Then you do an intense interval workout for thirty minutes, revving your heart rate, breathing, body temperature, hormone levels, and your metabolism. For up to seventy-two hours after you exercise, you'll be burning more calories than before. You may sit back down after your workout and burn 120 calories in that first hour, and 100 calories in the second hour. Tack that on to the calories you burn during the actual workout and you can start to see why intervals are so good for weight and fat loss.

The Workout

Intervals are part work, part recovery. When you're starting out, your recovery portions are going to be a lot longer than your periods of work. You may sprint for one minute then gently jog for two or three minutes. As you improve, your work periods may get a little shorter, and your rest periods may get a little longer because you learn to push yourself harder. The more conditioned you are, the easier it will be for you to catch your breath, feel your heart rate come back down, and feel prepared to give it your all again.

You can customize your own sprint and recover routine or choose one option from below.

Option 1: 30-second intervals at Level 10 (Sprint Interval Training, SIT)

Perform a thirty-second sprint interval at an "all-out" intensity (Intensity Level 10), followed by a four-minute recovery at Intensity Level 2. Repeat seven times.

NOTE: This would be written as 7 X 30 seconds:4 minutes, indicating seven sets of "all-out" exercise for thirty seconds followed by a four-minute recovery.

Option 2: 60-second intervals at Level 9
(High Intensity Interval Training, HIIT)

Perform a sixty-second sprint interval at an "almost all-out" intensity (Intensity Level 9), followed by a two-minute recovery at Intensity Level 2. Repeat nine times.

NOTE: This would be written as 9 X 60 seconds:2 minutes, indicating nine sets of "almost all-out" exercise for sixty seconds followed by a two-minute recovery.

You will want to start and end each interval workout with a warm-up and a cool-down. At the beginning and end of each interval session, perform a five-minute dynamic warm-up. After you're done with the complete round of intervals, finish your workout with a gentle cool-down stretch session. (See the Resistance Training chapter for complete instructions on the dynamic warm-up and cool-down sections.) Each complete interval workout will take between thirty and forty minutes.

When broken down by time, this is what Option 1 looks like:

0:00 to 5:00: Dynamic warm-up (see Resistance Training chapter for complete instructions)

5:00 to 5:30: Sprint at Intensity Level 10

5:30 to 9:00: Recover at Intensity Level 2

9:00 to 9:30: Sprint at Intensity Level 10

9:30 to 13:30: Recover at Intensity Level 2

13:30 to 14:00: Sprint at Intensity Level 10

14:00 to 17:00: Recover at Intensity Level 2

17:00 to 17:30: Sprint at Intensity Level 10

17:30 to 21:00: Recover at Intensity Level 2

21:00 to 21:30: Sprint at Intensity Level 10

21:30 to 25:00: Recover at Intensity Level 2

25:00 to 25:30: Sprint at Intensity Level 10

25:30 to 29:30: Recover at Intensity Level 2

29:30 to 30:00: Sprint at Intensity Level 10

30:00 to 32:00: Recover at Intensity Level 2

32:00 to 35:00: Gentle cool-down

Here is a chart of the interval workout options:

Interval Training (I) - Option I

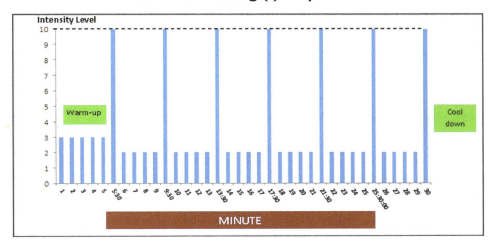

Interval Training (I) - Option 2

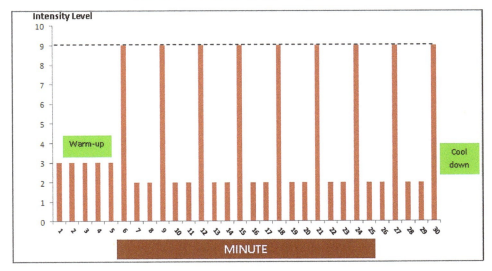

Intervals are an intense exercise routine, so be careful not to overdo it. Allow at least four days between interval sessions, and I recommend you perform each RISE routine one day per week for a total of four days of exercise per week. However, after the first four weeks of starting, feel free to choose one of the RISE routines to perform a second time, but I recommend not to exceed five days of exercise per week because your body needs time to recover, replenish, and rebuild. Always perform the dynamic warm-up before and a gentle cool-down after each session. Remember, this is always about work, then recovery. However, the great news is that recovery has new meaning because just think, with the "afterburn" working for you—instead of against you, when you go to relax—you will be burning more calories, even up to as long as seventy-two hours, than you would have if you had not done your interval training. That's motivation right there!

As stated above, this exercise routine has been scientifically proven to strengthen your heart, burn body fat, build muscle, and increase your metabolic rate (burn more calories) leading to improved overall health. It is also one of the most time-efficient forms of exercise you can perform. I know these days are so hectic that many of us are sprinting through life, but that is not the long-term answer. By taking these targeted sprints and resting when needed, we will win the race of a long, healthy, vital, and productive life. After all, I want you to *enjoy* the scenery of your life, and not *be* the scenery as the quote says!

12

S-STRETCHING—The Glue that Holds the Body Together

R
I

Stretching

E

Develop flexibility and you will be firm;
cultivate yielding and you will be strong.
—Liezi, *The Book of Master Lie*

During a recent television interview to discuss health and wellness, one of the producers asked me what I thought about stretching and yoga exercises. Interestingly, this is the most common exercise and fitness question I am asked, and my reply is always the same: Stretching, flexibility, and yoga is the "glue" that holds the body together, and without it, your body would fall apart and the risk of injury would increase dramatically.

Our muscular and skeletal (bones) systems function like pulleys and levers; therefore, they need to be kept well-lubricated and aligned properly. In addition, our tendons and muscles (the cables of the pulley) need to be adequately stretched and cared for to prevent them from becoming stiff and brittle to avoid tearing. Stretching exercises are particularly important the more physically active we are and as we age. A regular stretching/flexibility routine that moves the joints, tendons, ligaments, and muscles through a range of motion is critical to maintaining optimal health and function. This type of exercise routine may take different forms, such as simple stretching, yoga, qigong, Tai Chi, and Pilates, but the important point is it needs to be done consistently on a regular weekly basis.

Stretching can be done a lot of different ways, but my favorite is through yoga. I actually trained to get my yoga teaching certifications a few years ago because it seemed like the perfect complement to the other more intense types of exercise I did. Stretching and practicing yoga poses, or asanas, can increase flexibility, balance, and muscle tone and give you a greater sense of tranquility and peacefulness. Yoga also improves mobility while reducing blood sugar and belly fat and improving heart health and mood. Have trouble touching your toes? Not for long! On this program exercisers saw their hamstring flexibility improve by more than four inches, and they felt a lot more relaxed in stressful situations. Who doesn't want that?

Stretching is also restorative training because it improves balance, muscle tone, and flexibility, but it can lower blood sugar and even enhance mood. There are two main types of stretching/flexibility exercises you need to follow:

1) Static and 2) Dynamic

Static stretches are your quintessential stretches. You find a position that tests your flexibility, and then you hold it. This type of stretching usually involves holding a specific stretch for ten seconds or longer. Static stretching should be done only when the muscles are warm and there is increased blood flow and circulation. This will enhance recovery from physical exercise training as well as reduce injury, because it properly stretches the muscles and helps enhance blood flow and removal of waste products. Static stretching is best performed as a confined "Stretching" exercise routine or after you've performed resistance, interval or endurance exercise. You may have heard that you should reserve five to ten minutes for static stretching *after* you have exercised. That's the perfect time to do it since your muscles will be plenty warm, and stretching can actually improve your recovery from the hard work. However, you can also perform this type of stretching during some workouts, such as yoga, Pilates, and Tai Chi.

Dynamic stretches are active movements. Swinging, sweeping, twisting, and stepping. Dynamic stretching means moving through various ranges of motion, not just holding one position. These are often used as warm-up exercises.

Dynamic stretching will enhance physical performance and muscle action as well as reduce injury, because it prepares the muscles for movement by activating (think awakening) the nerves and muscles fibers. Warming up the muscles prior to stretching or movement increases the delivery of vital oxygen and nutrients to the muscles, which are necessary to provide movement. (Cue up the image of pro athletes getting warmed up before a big game.) Dynamic stretches are active in nature. You move continuously through a full range of motion in an attempt to "wake up" or activate your muscles, tendons, ligaments, and bones so you are absolutely ready to perform whatever sport or activity you're preparing for.

RISE with Stretching

Who has time for stretching? You should, if you want your body to perform at its peak. I get it. All you want to do is move, to feel like you're really shedding pounds, zapping calories, and building strength. But integrating stretching or stretch-based workouts such as yoga will actually benefit your other workouts. Stretching, flexibility, and yoga are the "glue" that holds the body together. Without it, your body wouldn't function as well, and the risk of injury would increase dramatically.

Stretching brings four types of balance to the body. It can add length to muscles that are getting stronger and shorter. This is important because most athletes benefit from a large range of motion. (There are, of course, some exceptions where tight muscles can help your performance, but unless you're an Olympic hopeful, you probably don't need to worry about this.) Stretching can also address imbalances in the body, creating symmetry, stability, and better form. If a swimmer has one flexible shoulder and one tight one, they aren't going to cover the length of the pool as quickly or easily if their range of motion was equal. Finally, the toned-down energy required during stretching or yoga is a good counter to workouts such as intervals. You're moving some—enough to relieve delayed onset muscle soreness and increase your circulation—but not enough to tire you out. In fact, you might even feel like you're taking a rest day, which is a must for proper maintenance. There's even a fourth way stretching can help with balance. Stretching—at least in the form of yoga poses—can help you improve your actual balance as you learn to hold precarious poses without wobbling or wiggling. But my favorite reason to practice stretching exercises and yoga poses is because it naturally increases mood and lowers anxiety by elevating brain levels of the neurotransmitter gamma-aminobutyric acid (GABA).[75] This finding alone should have you running out to buy a yoga mat and then get started with my PRISE stretching routine! Most conventional pharmacological medications/drugs prescribed with the goal of improving mood and lowering anxiety aim to increase GABA levels, but usually always are accompanied by side effects. Stretching and yoga may provide the same benefits but without the side effects.

As with everything else I suggest in this book, I really practice what I preach. As a certified yoga instructor in two different forms, I've led thousands of people through yoga workouts—from CEOs to top athletes. I also regularly do my own yoga workouts. I've found it's the best way for me to enhance my muscle flexibility and joint mobility and at the same time reconnect my mind to my body. My favorite time to do my **Stretching** routine is after a strenuous **Resistance, Interval** or **Endurance** workout the day before. In this plan, you only need to do one sixty-minute stretching workout each week. But if you find you like to do more—waking up with five minutes of yoga or fitting in a few stretching poses in the afternoon—I actually encourage you to do so. Unlike the other type of trainings in the RISE program, it's quite hard to overdo stretching.

Stretching 101

If the body is a machine, the muscles and tendons function like its pulleys and cables. They need to be well-lubricated and aligned to move smoothly. They also need to be adequately stretched and cared for to prevent stiffness, brittleness, or tearing. Stretching can do all of this. Although flexibility work is important for everyone, its especially necessary as we become more physically active and as we age.

A regular stretching and flexibility routine moves the joints, tendons, ligaments, and muscles through a maximum range of motion. You can practice this many different ways, from the simple stretching you might do after a run or in a class such as yoga, Tai Chi, or Pilates. At its root, stretching is simply gentle and mindful movement. The type of stretching you do is actually less important than the regularity with which you do it. In order for stretching to be effective, you must do it consistently on a regular weekly basis.

75   Chris C. Streeter et al., *Journal of Alternative and Complementary Medicine*, November 2010. Accessed March 20, 2018. https://www.ncbi.nlm.nih.gov/pmc/articles/PMC3111147/.

When you stretch you may feel a small tug in your muscles. Or you might simply feel your joints warming and opening. Both of these results can come from stretching, although they are likely the by-product of the two different types of stretching and flexibility exercises: dynamic stretching and static stretching.

The Workout

The stretching routine in this program involves traditional yoga poses called "asanas" with a combination of core and strengthening elements for a total body workout that will leave you rejuvenated and recharged. I have included some sample pictures in appendix D; however, I do have and an exercise journal and handbook available that is more comprehensive.

Warm-up Stretches (Sun Salutations):
    1) Mountain Pose (Tadasana)
    2) Standing Forward Bend (Uttanasana)
    3) Plank Pose (Phalakasana)
    4) Four-Limbed Staff Pose (Chaturanga Dandasana)
    5) Cobra Pose (Bhujangasana)
    6) Upward Facing Dog Pose (Urdhva Mukha Svanasana)
    7) Downward Facing Dog Pose (Adha Mukha Svanasana)
    8) Child's Pose/Rest Pose (Balasana)

Standing Stretches:
    1) Neck Stretching
    2) Side Bending
    3) Lunge Pose (Anjaneyasana)
    4) Warrior I Pose (Virabhadrasana I)
    5) Warrior II Pose (Virabhadrana II)
    6) Triangle Pose (Utthita Trikonasana)
    7) Extended Side Angle Pose (Utthita Parsvakonasana)
    8) Goddess Pose (Utkata Konasana)
    9) Chair Pose (Utkatasana)
    10) Revolved Chair Pose (Parivrtta Utkatasana)

11) Squat Pose (Malasana)

12) Standing Wide-Legged Forward Bend Pose (Prasarita Padottanasana)

Balance in Motion Stretches:

1) Tree Pose (Vrksasana)

2) Warrior III (Virabhadrasana III)

3) Lord of the Dance Pose (Natarajasana

4) Standing One-Legged Balance

5) Eagle Pose (Garudasana)

6) Boat Pose (Navasana)

7) Bicycle Pose

8) Bow Pose (Dhanurasana)

9) Candlestick Pose

10) Camel Pose (Ustrasana)

11) Pigeon Pose (Eke Pada Rajakapotasana)

Floor Stretches:

1) Seated Cross-Legged Pose (Sukhasana)

2) Staff Pose (Dandasana)

3) Seated Forward Bend (Paschimottanasana)

4) Head to Knee Pose (Janu Sirsasana)

5) Wide Seated Forward Bend Pose (Upavistha Konasana)

6) Table Top Pose & Cat/Cow

7) Bridge Pose (Setu Bandhasana)

8) Extended Puppy Dog Pose (Uttana Shishosana)

9) Butterfly Pose (Baddha Konasana)

10) Happy Baby Pose (Ananda Balasana)

11) Half Twist Pose (Ardha Matsyendrasana)

12) Head to Knee Pose (Janu Sirsasana)

13) Front Split Pose (Hanumanasana)

14) Frog Pose (Mandukasana)

15) Spinal Twist Pose (Supta Matsyendrasana)

16) Corpse Pose (Savasana)

17) Reclining Bound Angle Pose (Supta Baddha Konasana)

If you stretch in a gentle but regular way, you'll gradually open up your muscles, making it easier to exercise and also increasing your ability to do everyday things, like reaching for items on the top shelf or picking up things off the floor and maintaining your balance on uneven or slippery surfaces. Of course, if you don't take stretching seriously or don't try to push yourself a little more each time you reach for your toes or open your arms wide, you won't see many changes. On the other hand, if you push yourself way into the uncomfortable zone, you may be able to touch your toes, but you may get there by tearing your hamstring or otherwise injuring yourself. To find that middle ground, I encourage people to bring the stretch to the "soft edge, that place where you feel the tightness in the muscle but you bring your awareness and your breath to the tightness and then breathe past it. This is a really cool place to be because it heightens your awareness and mindfulness of your body. In a short time, you may be enjoying yourself so much that you want to commit more than one day a week to it! It's a great stress-buster and mood enhancer, so of all the exercise routines one can safely add extras to my protocol.

Stretching creates flexibility, pliability, and mobility, and these create strength and power and keep you injury-free. The amazing thing is that is not only true of our muscles but of our emotions and mind-set. People who can't face change or who are inflexible (unpliable) cause themselves to suffer in more ways than necessary. They create an energy around them that makes it difficult to grow or to find deep peace and understanding of others. Every day is such a gift that if we allow our minds to grow, to be flexible, if we work it like our muscles, if we stretch ourselves and our beliefs, we will discover the world and people have so much more to offer. It is why the great masters who have lived and taught us through the centuries have had so many answers to the baffling questions we struggle with about the universe. When you think about what Liezi teaches when he says, "*Develop flexibility and you will be firm; cultivate yielding and you will be strong*," understand that this goes much deeper than the muscles themselves. And one day, hopefully soon, I will teach you about the practice of integrative health and the importance of turning inward to master the world around us.

13

E-ENDURANCE—Nature's Aphrodisiac a.k.a. the Runner's "High"

Endurance

Diamonds are nothing more than chunks of coal that stuck to their jobs.
—Malcom Stevenson Forbes

Yes, diamonds are proof of endurance! Don't worry, I'm not asking *that* much of you, and whether we agree with the *Forbes* fortune or not, they stuck to their jobs. In the fitness world, endurance is another name for what a lot of people refer to as cardiovascular or aerobic exercise—those long and continuous jogs, walks, swims, or bike rides. Doing exercise like this for an hour or more is one of the surest ways to help lower blood pressure and blood sugar, both of which reduce your risk for heart disease and type 2 diabetes. This type of exercise also includes running, swimming, hiking, cross-country skiing, snowshoeing, rollerblading, and rowing, among other sports. Endurance exercise is good for your body, and it also has a tremendous effect on brain health, including enhanced cognition, brain function, and feelings of happiness. It can also help reduce feelings of depression, tension, and anxiety. People talk about the "runner's high," but it can really come from any type of continuous endurance activity.

Several years ago, I read a fascinating research study from Germany that documented the runner's high in humans, for the first time.[76] By definition,

---

76   H. Boecker et al., "The runners high: opioidergic mechanisms in the human brain." Cerebral cortex (New York, N.Y.: 1991), November 2008. Accessed March 20, 2018. https://www.ncbi.nlm.nih.gov/pubmed/18296435.

the runner's high is an enhanced mood state that occurs during or following endurance exercise of more than an hour. It is related to a flood of endorphins in the brain, which are associated with feelings of euphoria, happiness, and for some, extreme peacefulness. The more endorphins released during exercise, the more intense the feelings.

Up until this study, the runner's high was mostly anecdotal and never actually proven to exist from a scientific standpoint. However, the findings provided firsthand evidence that exercise ($\geq$ 60 minutes) increases endorphin release in the brain as well as feelings of euphoria and happiness.

As an avid endurance athlete myself, I have experienced the runner's high for decades, so this study validated that my feelings were not imagined. More importantly, the study proved that the runner's high is real, and performing endurance exercise increases feelings of euphoria, happiness, and peacefulness—it's the purest form of a natural high. Endurance exercise can be addictive because of the runner's high.

One of my favorite side effects of endurance exercise is the opportunity to experience synchrony among all the different systems of the body, such as the beating of my heart, the rhythm of my breathing, and the contraction of my muscles, often referred to as *entrainment*. This occurs most commonly when you are performing endurance exercise and using your full body in a rhythmical movement pattern, such as jogging/running, cycling, or swimming, and your breathing, heartbeat, and muscle contractions all begin to work in synchrony. It's a beautiful occurrence when it happens, and I've experienced it often during my days as an endurance/triathlete. It's like a symphony, all the moving parts working together to create something much bigger than the individual parts. The same way each member of an orchestra can play beautiful music on their own, but when they all come together and perform as a whole the music comes alive even more. This is what happens when we perform endurance training using *entrainment*. The heartbeat, lungs, muscles, and nervous system are each capable of supporting the exercise independently of each other; however, when they are working synchronously, the result is magnificent—exercise becomes almost effortless, tremendously enjoyable, almost meditative and spiritual in nature.

This is the goal of the Endurance exercise routine, to become transformative and to bring you to another dimension of self-awareness/actualization. I like to perform the endurance routine out in nature and first thing in the morning because it's so serene, peaceful, and quiet and the body is still relatively silent, and at 60%–70% intensity, it results in the greatest brain blood flow and most likely setting for a euphoric runner's high and mood boost!

If you're intimidated by the idea of endurance activity—or exercising continuously for an hour or more—let that feeling go. All of you reading this are capable of performing an endurance routine using the guidelines I provide. Indeed, you probably already do some sort of endurance training, whether it's in the form of walking up and down the aisles of the grocery store, playing in a recreational soccer game, or heading out on an afternoon hike or swimming some laps. All continuous activity counts, even if it's gentle movement. Of course, for the maximum benefits, the intensity needs to be such that you're at least a little breathless.

Endurance 101

Endurance exercise includes any type of activity that engages the majority of your body mass. This means walking, jogging, running, cycling, swimming, hiking, cross-country skiing, snowshoeing, rollerblading, rowing, dancing, and more. Of course, you can do all of these activities as intervals or as short workouts. To make sure you're training to effectively increase your endurance, you must keep going for an hour or longer.

What's so important about sixty minutes (or more) of activity? By exercising for this amount of time, you begin to illuminate receptors in your brain that are associated with feelings of euphoria and happiness, which ultimately leads to the "natural high" people experience while engaged in endurance exercise. This is much more likely to happen while we are outside in the naturalistic environment of the outdoors in nature.

Knowing what's happening in your body may be enough to get you out for your weekly endurance workout. But if you need more convincing, learning about the runner's high should do the trick. By definition, the runner's high is an enhanced mood state that occurs during or after endurance exercise of more than an hour. It can be a result of running, swimming, cycling, or any other type of activity. (The name "runner's high" is a bit of a misnomer.) This joyful feeling is the result of a flood of the endorphins in the brain. Endorphins are chemicals released by the body during a handful of activities, including extreme or thrill-seeking sports like sky diving, rock climbing, heli-skiing, endurance exercise, laughter, and sex. They're often called "feel-good chemicals," since they block feelings of stress or pain. Endorphins are associated with feelings of euphoria, happiness, and even extreme peacefulness. The more endorphins are released during exercise, the more intense the feelings.

As an avid endurance athlete, I've experienced the runner's high for decades. I wouldn't go so far as to say that I'm addicted to endurance exercise, but I fit in at least one session each week. This feeling of the runner's high is one main reason. If you ask me, it's the purest form of euphoria and bliss.

With endurance work, the formula is still the same. You're going to schedule a sixty-minute or longer endurance exercise session each week. Even if you're an absolute beginner, you can keep going for a full hour. Just focus on starting slow and slightly increasing your speed each time. You may start walking and build up to simply walking with more intensity, something you can accomplish by increasing your speed, finding a place to walk that has a slight incline so you're walking uphill, and even by pumping your arms more vigorously. Remember, only achieve a level 6 on my Intensity scale.

Dr. Paul's PRISE Tips for Endurance Fitness:

As you get moving, keep these tips in mind:

◊ **Aim for an Intensity Level of 6 out of 10.** What does a six feel like? This is a level of activity where you can have a conversation with a friend for hours. You may be breathing a little heavy, but you can still spit out full sentences and even paragraphs of dialogue.

◊ **Get out in nature.** Studies show that going out into the woods, a grassy field, or even a park can make you feel even happier and more revitalized. (Of course, if you fire up the treadmill on days when there's bad weather, you may feel even better being inside!)

◊ **Move first thing in the morning.** Just like the stretching workout, I'd recommend you do this right after getting out of bed, either before you have eaten (I call this "Fasted Endurance" others may refer to it as "Fasted Cardio") or after a small morning snack. Make sure you take a moment to first hydrate with water, tea, or a little morning java without cream and sugar. The Fasted Endurance routine has really caught on recently, especially for those interested in losing weight and body fat. I've experimented with this myself and found it to be a mildly effective strategy to accelerate body fat loss if done properly. Here are my recommendations and cautions of Fasted Endurance: 1) Aim for a maximum of sixty minutes per session at Intensity Level 6 or 7; 2) Perform no more than one time per week; 3) make sure to replenish, refuel, and rehydrate with electrolytes (sodium, potassium, magnesium, chloride, calcium) during and after along with 20–40 g of high-quality protein within two hours of finishing the workout. It's super important to follow these guidelines for Fasted Endurance to maximize the fat burning, maintain adequate hydration and muscle function, and minimize lean muscle mass loss that commonly occurs with repeated or inappropriate Fasted Endurance. I want to let you in on a little secret: "Fasted Core" is a much more effective fitness routine to "shred abs" and burn belly fat than "Fasted Endurance." I explain this in depth in my next book *The PRISE Protocol Training Manual* so keep a look out for this in the near future!

◊ **Refuel as needed.** If you plan to exercise for more than sixty minutes, bring along extra nourishment, just in case. You might find you prefer a sports drink with electrolytes, a small packet of trail mix, or an energy gel. After one hour of moving, your body and brain may need this extra fuel to keep going strong.

◊ **Ditch the distractions.** You may want to scroll past this suggestion, but I would strongly recommend you exercise without any electronic devices, except maybe a watch or heart rate monitor. That means no music, no TV, no checking email. (For you old-schoolers, no paper books or magazines either!) This will allow you to "tune in" to your own body rhythms, feeling and listening to your body's feedback as you exercise. Noticing your breath, heart rate, and the general feeling of effort you're putting out can help you decide to speed up, slow down, or otherwise change your workout. This is called being mindful and present with your body, and it is one surefire way to become a better athlete.

The Workout

At the beginning of each endurance session, remember to perform that <u>five-minute dynamic warm-up and a gentle stretch when you finish</u>. Use any mode

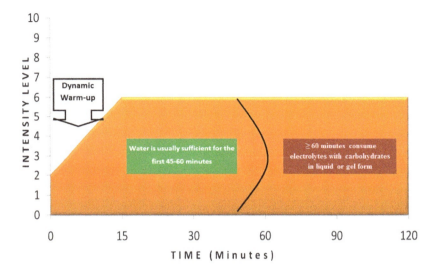

of exercise that uses the majority of your body (swimming, walking, running, cycling, cross-country skiing, rollerblading, skating, snowshoeing, hiking, etc.).

Another note about endurance and a winning combination: it is getting this endurance outdoors in the real, *outdoor* air and learning to just breathe! To follow my theme about the importance of Mother Nature, I want to expand on the truth about solitude endurance exercise in nature itself—not the gym. For those of you who know me, you know that I am a huge proponent of performing most of your physical exercise outdoors in nature so you can truly disconnect from your wired world and connect to your inner world. By your inner world I am, of course, referring to the harmony of you: spirit, mind, and body.

While I fully understand, appreciate, and have even proven through scientific research that performing exercise while virtually engaged with an interactive video game (called "exergaming")[77] is beneficial for our brain health in

---

[77] The study that has received an enormous amounts of media attention in things such as *O Magazine*, *Time*, and others:

    C. Anderson-Hanley, P. J. Arciero, A. M. Brickman, J. P. Nimon, N. Okuma, S. C. Westen, M. E.

certain circumstances, I also believe that exercising outdoors in nature has supe-rior health benefits compared to indoor exercise. The best news is there is now scientific evidence to support my belief.

Researchers from Peninsula College of Medicine and Dentistry in the UK analyzed data from 833 adults and showed that mental well-being was improved while exercising outdoors in nature compared to exercising indoors. Some of the health benefits included increased energy, feelings of engagement, joy, and satisfaction, along with decreased tension, confusion, anger, and depression.

This leads me to my next point. I have consistently urged people to perform endurance exercise outdoors in nature as a way to improve their psychological well-being and not necessarily as a weight-loss strategy. Fortunately, these cur-rent research findings support my hunch. When you exercise outdoors, you will likely "think" and "feel" better, which may lead to making better lifestyle choices or "actions." Therefore, instead of using endurance exercise to help burn more calories, focus on the improved mood state effects that may result and may lead to healthy lifestyle choices, such as choosing higher quality foods to nourish your body. In fact, there is evidence that endurance exercise may actually pro-mote food intake, making it harder to curb your appetite. But by performing endurance exercise outdoors in nature, it may offset the increased food intake by enhancing your mood, leading to better food choices.

Of course, my research, and that of other scientists, has also shown that endurance exercise is very beneficial for improving your body's ability to me-tabolize sugar in your blood and help lower your blood pressure, two extremely important health benefits that drastically reduce your risk for heart disease and diabetes. The bottom line is that you need to adopt the understanding that per-forming endurance exercise outside in nature extends beyond the calories you burn while doing it and instead improves your overall mood state and reduces your risk for heart disease and diabetes. So, get up from the couch and make an appointment with Mother Nature today!

It's wonderful to know that with this type of activity, aside from the pride of knowing your body is strong enough to go-go-go for an hour or more, is that you are helping prevent your body from illness and premature aging. How

Merz, B. D. Pence, J. A. Woods, A. F. Kramer, and E. A. Zimmerman. "Exergaming and older adult cognition: a cluster randomized clinical trial." *American Journal of Preventive Medicine*. February 2012. Accessed March 20, 2018. https://www.ncbi.nlm.nih.gov/pubmed/22261206.

exciting to know it burns major calories and positively increases brain health, including enhanced cognition, brain function, and mood state. In layman's terms, this means you might find you have an easier time remembering things, solving problems, and managing stress all day long! As a bonus, at the end of long bout of endurance activity, you might get a huge burst of happiness—Mother Nature's aphrodisiac or "runner's high." In this case, it's Dr. Paul approved!

14

Food Is Thy Medicine:
Time it Like You Time Your Meds

Ancient Egyptian proverb: "One-quarter of what you eat keeps you alive. The other three-quarters keeps your doctor alive."

We have probably all heard the Hypocrites quote: "Let food be thy medicine." Well, there is one other fact that I am going to add: Pick the right ones and then *time* them properly. I spent enough time on protein and Protein Pacing and now I just want to come back quickly to fats. Remember how I spoke about the fat-adapted Protein Pacing as allowing even more chances to lose weight and grow lean muscle? Well, I am referring to specific and healthy types of fats.

Here is a general breakdown of the fats to love, and where to find them:

Fats to love:

Specific Saturated fats: Highly stable, largely non-reactive molecules with a good shelf life. These are generally solid at room temperature.

◊ Butter from grass-fed cows: An excellent source of fat-soluble vitamins A, D, and K, butter from certified 100% grass-fed cows is not always available year round but can be recognized by the distinctive golden yellow color obtained through the presence of naturally occurring beta-carotene, a powerful antioxidant. Butter from grass-fed cows also contains conjugated-linoleic acid (CLA), which may have anti-cancer properties.[78] Short-chain fatty acids are easily and quickly absorbed

---

78 Mian M. K. Shahzad et al., "Trans10, cis12 conjugated linoleic acid inhibits proliferation and migration of ovarian cancer cells by inducing ER stress, autophagy, and modulation of Src," PLOS ONE, January 11, 2018. Accessed February 23, 2018. http://paperity.org/p/85521415/trans10-cis12-conjugated-linoleic-acid-inhibits-proliferation-and-migration-of-ovarian.

through the GI tract where they are immediately metabolized for energy in healthy active people. [79]

◊ Coconut oil:

Largely made up of short- and medium-chain fatty acids

Antimicrobial properties

Can be kept at room temperature for a long time without rancidity.

◊ Lauric acid:

Found in cow and goat milk, palm kernal oil

Limit to 10-20 grams per day

Monounsaturated fats: These fats are found in foods like almonds, olive oil, and avocados. They are slightly less stable than saturated fats, and so are often liquid at room temperature.

Polyunsaturated fats: These fats are generally considered the most unstable. They are made up of long carbon chains that do not "stack" together well. This means that they are often liquid even below room temperature. These oils are susceptible to spoilage (rancidity) and can easily burn or oxidize when used as a cooking agent. For this reason, it's usually not a good idea to use polyunsaturated fats while cooking.

Just as essential to being successful with PRISE is the timing, so here are some more tips:

Listen to what your body is telling you (listen to body cues).

As I've highlighted numerous times in the book, counting and measuring your calories is not nearly as healthy and beneficial for your overall health as the quality and timing of your calories. In other words, the quality of your calories always reigns supreme over the quantity of your calories for optimal health and peak performance. With this in mind, the number one question I'm bombarded with on a daily basis from my followers and others is, "Which specific nutrition plan (diet) should I be following for the best results?" My answer is always the same. "The best nutrition plan is the one your body tells you to eat!"

---

79 M. Bugaut, "Occurrence, Absorption and Metabolism of Short Chain Fatty Acids in the Digestive Tract of Mammals," Comparative Biochemistry and Physiology. B, Comparative Biochemistry. Accessed March 5, 2018, https://www.ncbi.nlm.nih.gov/pubmed/3297476.

This response usually comes with a bit of a perplexed and confused look by the person, so then I have to explain a bit further. Our bodies are programmed for "homeostasis," which means a state of equilibrium among cellular and overall physiological processes that maintain a balanced resting (normal) state. When things are "off" in our bodies, signals are sent from our cells, tissues, organs, etc. to our brains in an attempt to correct the problem. Within the context of optimal nourishment for health and performance, the same thing happens. If we are depleted of essential nutrients, our bodies will send warning signals to the brain to increase our intake of those nutrients. One nutrient that is top priority every day is our protein stores, because proteins are involved in every cellular process of the body and can never be compromised. This is why Protein Pacing is a necessity and foundation for EVERY type of diet and nutrition plan. But when it comes to fats and carbs, they can wax and wane on a daily basis, depending on the needs of the body (cells).

My advice is as follows: If you crave carb foods, this means you may likely be lacking in vitamins, minerals and fiber and therefore should increase your intake of fresh vegetables, fruits, legumes (beans), and whole grains. Whereas, if you are craving more fatty foods, you're probably exhausted (physically and emotionally), maybe more prone to sickness and need the additional calories from foods like avocados, nuts, seeds, and oils (coconut, olive, etc.) to help replenish your energy stores and fuel your nervous and immune systems, which depends on a healthy dose of essential fats/lipids (fatty acids) for optimal function. Listening to your body and what it's telling you is proof there is no single best diet for anyone. We need to adapt and be nimble on a daily basis with the foundation of ALL nutrition plans being Protein Pacing! I hope by now, it has become crystal clear why Protein Pacing needs to be the core form of nourishment at each meal for the rest of your life and with carbs and fats included as needed.

Eat more often with Protein Pacing. You may have heard that eating at timed-intervals throughout the day burns more calories than aiming for three square meals. But for years there wasn't much actual evidence to support this. Then I drafted one of the first studies to show that frequent mini-meals—especially those containing high-quality, lean protein—raise metabolism, burn more calories, and zap more belly fat than three meals a day. This doesn't mean grazing and snacking all day but instead aim for four to six high-quality Protein Pacing meals and snacks throughout the day evenly spaced every 3-4 hours.

How exactly does this eat-more, lose-more approach work? The trick is to keep your metabolism revved continuously with these Protein Pacing meals. You can do this by paying attention to the amount and type of protein foods you're eating and how you're spacing your meals throughout the day. The goal from this style of eating is to provide the body with the ideal amount and type of high-quality protein to fuel the cells of the body so they can maximize the pathway of protein synthesis every few hours instead of overloading your system with too large a load of protein with just a few meals a day. If weight loss is your goal, you may find it's easiest to simply cut your current meals in half—literally—eating one half in one sitting and the other half a few hours later but making sure your protein intake is at the critical amount of 20–40 g. I usually advise people to eat four to six times a day.

If you've been worried that eating more often might spell trouble for your diet, think again. One of my favorite things about this pacing approach is that you're less likely to give in to cravings. Research shows you feel fuller on small, frequent protein-balanced meals than after eating a few big meals. A lot of the people I've worked with say their extra calories come from the unexpected snacks they take in throughout the day. The cookie they grab from the office break room or the soda they reach for when they start to feel a little sluggish in the afternoon (I'm sure you know exactly what I mean). When you actually plan in these small and frequent "protein-pacing" food breaks, you're much less likely to eat off script and eat unhealthy things. And there's one more benefit to smaller portions spaced out throughout the day: no more bloat or feeling of being "stuffed"!

I recommend you eat throughout the day using my Protein Pacing plan. But what about the night? My mother used to say that no good things ever happened after midnight. With eating, I'd venture it's more like 8:00 p.m. Setting this cutoff for yourself will eliminate the calories that come from late-night crunching and munching, and it'll also give your metabolism a chance to really rest before the next day. Plus, the calories you eat at night are more likely to be stored as fat rather than burned off, so limit your intake after dinner to my Bedtime Bellyfat Burner (BBB) plan, which is the last snack of the day. This is actually one of the most important snacks of the day (other than my Morning Muscle Maximizer, MMM) because it provides a high-quality protein feeding during the overnight time period, which fuels and feeds your muscles so you can burn fat throughout the night. How does this sound? You can have the occasional glass of wine or beer with your evening meal if you like, but switch to water or herbal tea after that. But no matter what, make the last calories you eat a Protein Pacing snack of 20–30 g of high-quality protein.

Dish out more low-energy nutrient-dense (LEND) foods. Protein isn't the only thing I want you to eat more of, high-fiber should also be on the list. There are a ton of foods that are filling without being heavy. These foods can help you get the nutrients you need to stay healthy and strong, but they won't make you pack on pounds. In fact, they'll do just the opposite. You can eat a plateful of these low-energy nutrient-dense (LEND) foods and lose weight because they're not full of calories. These LEND foods will supply vitamins, minerals, fiber, and special nutrients called phytochemicals (plant chemicals), which fight disease and increase energy levels but don't carry a high caloric cost.

LEND foods tend to be high in fiber, which keeps you regular, lowers cholesterol, maintains blood sugar levels, and can make you feel full. Just like protein, these LEND foods require more energy to digest and metabolize than a lot of other foods. That means you can eat more without worrying about those bites sticking to your belly, hips, and thighs.

If you've been worried the Protein Pacing plan will tell you to eat plain chicken breasts all day long, my LEND list will put those fears to rest. All plant-based foods such as green and rainbow-colored fresh vegetables and fruits are LEND foods, and so are legumes, such as lentils, split peas, chickpeas, black beans, and kidney beans. You can also go nuts over nuts and seeds like chia, pumpkin (pepitas), and flaxseed and whole grains such as quinoa, oats, barley, and rice. I've already talked about protein-rich foods like lean meats, but they're on the LEND list too.

Having shared all of the above, I want to make sure I tell you that there is some truth to those additional calories, and here is my tip that gets me as close to a "dieting" plan as I feel comfortable with:

Shave off surplus calories. So, just how much of these foods do you get to eat? If your goal is weight loss and you're into calorie counting, I'd aim for about 1200–1400 calories a day for women and 1500–1800 calories a day for men. Right now, you may eat only a few hundred calories more than this, consuming more like 1800–2000 calories a day. Stopping at 1200–1800 calories will be easy if you follow my five other tips.

Keep in mind, I don't want you to ever feel hungry or deprived. You may eat the same volume of food—or an even greater amount—but the foods you eat will have more metabolically active nutrients (protein) and fewer calories in them. You may go from eating a few slices of pizza to eating a salad with chicken and a side of hummus and pita. Your belly will be happy, but you won't be storing all those excess calories as fat. If you have pounds to lose, it's an indication that you may have been eating the wrong amount, types, and timing of foods for your body to burn and instead stored those extra calories in your trouble zones—usually the hips, thighs, and belly.

Once you've mastered this style of eating, you might want to try cutting out more surplus calories. In some of my recent studies, when women and men followed this same eating plan just at 1200 and 1500 calories a day, respectively, weight loss results skyrocketed to an average of 25 pounds in 11 weeks, or about 2.5 months. Of course, if you're in a hurry to meet your weight-loss goals, you can jump right in and start here. You already have the tools—the LEND list, the Protein Pacing, the reduction of processed foods and carbohydrates—so follow the diet at the calorie count that best serves you. In general, eating slightly more calories of healthier food from a better source is always better than feeling deprived and seeking refuge in processed food. Give yourself some slack during your dietary transition if times get tough and you start to feel hungry. Fat- and protein-dense snacks such as an avocado with some wild fish or slices of free-range chicken or a protein shake/smoothie or bar can help to signal satiety and decrease any sugar cravings you may be having—a worthy goal even if it means you eat more calories than usual for that day.

Finally, never forget Grandma's cooking:

Eat home-cooked food that is grown locally or organic whenever possible. Shopping for, preparing, and cooking your own food is one easy way to cut calories. It may not seem like it, but a majority of the foods you eat regularly are probably highly processed foods—things like crackers and chips as well as high sodium packaged meals and sugary bottled drinks. Even at restaurants, a lot of the foods you eat are prepackaged and just heated up. True cooking is hard to come by outside of your kitchen, but it's important if you want to know what's actually going into your body.

There's another big problem with packaged foods: they're actually manufactured to make you feel hungrier after eating them, not full. Most processed foods contain the "big three": lots of fat, sugar, and salt, all of which trigger your hunger signals to fire at warp speed. Processed foods are designed in big laboratories with the intention of making it so that the more you eat, the more you want to eat. This happens because the foods are missing vital nutrients your body needs so they leave you hungry for more. By swapping out a bag of chips for a snack of an apple with nut or seed butter, you'll feel full for much longer without taking in any extra calories.

How do you do it when you're pressed for time? It's all about planning. My wife and I raised our three boys on home-cooked meals by making up a new menu each week and doing shopping and prep on the weekend, before homework and sports practices kicked into high gear. If chili was on the menu, I'd pre-chop all of my veggies as soon as I got home from the store. If we were having taco night, my wife would cook up extra ground turkey to be used in the next night's marinara sauce. Look for ways to get ahead, and cooking will feel a lot more manageable. Also, don't be afraid of using packaged foods like canned tomatoes or beans or frozen spinach and even protein powders (whey and plantbased) to add to baked goods, casseroles, soups or as on-the-go meals. As I mentioned earlier, avoid highly processed foods with too much salt, sugar, and unhealthy fat and instead take advantage of nutrient-dense engineered foods that come in the form of protein powders, bars and snacks. I've used these extensively in my research showing phenomenal benefits. These are a far cry from the pre-made macaroni and cheese microwave dinners I want you to eliminate. If you can swap in a few pre-cut, or pre-cooked ingredients into an otherwise fresh meal, I'm all for it!

Armed with the above tips, did all this information on food make you hungry? If it also feels a little overwhelming, I understand. These tips are pretty easy to follow, but you'll likely need to make a trip to a grocery store and chart out a few meals before you can really make it a regular part of your life. In this chapter, you'll find lists of my favorite protein sources as well as the LEND foods that will also take up a good part of your diet. I hope you're surprised at just how many types of food are on these lists. I want you to feel inspired to cook and eat and for the Protein-Pacing plan to be easy to follow. Thirty years of nutrition and metabolism research has taught me two main lessons:

1) Our bodies thrive on a diet consisting of 25% to 35% lean, healthy protein (from both plant and animal sources; roughly 20–40 g of protein per meal), along with at least 25% healthy fats and oils and lots of fresh veggies, certain whole grains, and fruits; and 2) Performing a combination of exercise routines, as opposed to just one or two different types, on a weekly basis results in drastic health and physical performance improvements.

Protein Pacing holds the key to weight loss. Several recent intervention studies from our laboratory provide strong support for eating a protein-rich diet—think a quarter to a third of your daily calories—to decrease total body weight and body fat (including abdominal fat) while improving cardiovascular and metabolic health. Our study diets range between 25% and 35% of high-quality animal- and plant-based protein that emphasize foods such as nuts/seeds, legumes, beans, pea/rice protein powder, free-range eggs, grass-fed dairy products (milk, Greek yogurt, cottage cheese, whey protein powder), wild fish, and grass-fed beef.

As a leader in health care, I believe we need to be more inclusive (not divisive) and promote a balanced nutritional eating landscape that doesn't alienate one food group from another. A balance of high-quality nutrient-dense whole foods from local and/or organic plant and animal sources are best for optimal health. Both animal and plant-based diets provide superior health benefits. We just need to focus on the "quality" of the source of each and find more harmony in our nutritional recommendations.

Quality of Your Proteins, Fats, and Carbs: Like almost anything consumable, not all available foods are created equal. While it is true that good food can be expensive in the moment, it is best to always minimize the toxins in your food while maximizing nutrition and health benefits from every item that enters your body. The most obvious argument in favor of more expensive food is that healthier people need to spend less money on health care in the future! Healthy, organic, local, humanely raised, small farm produce, meat, and dairy take more work to produce and are thus more expensive. This food is also better for you, it tastes better, and its purchase gives money back to your local communities. Not everyone has access to these resources but, whenever you can, endeavor to buy (in order of importance): Unprocessed/pure (no additives, just the thing you want!), organic (non-GMO and without chemicals or synthetic pesticides), and local food. If you must prioritize which foods to spend more money on, include meat, dairy, and eggs. In general, foods containing more fat store far more toxins than non-fatty foods do, making their quality of utmost importance. For example, scientific evidence has shown that grass-fed animal sources (beef, dairy, eggs, etc.) have a higher nutritional content and a much healthier fatty acid profile than factory-farmed animal sources, especially beef and the same goes for organic produce.

When you go to the grocery store, take this book so you can reference these important lists as you shop. These are many of the foods that are a staple in my diet and on the Protein Pacing plan.

Protein Pacing in Action:

You've read that protein is important for getting your metabolism going. On this plan, I recommend eating 20–40 g per sitting. This is the amount that will keep your body feeling full and properly fueled until your next mini-meal in a few hours.

Sources of Protein, , and CHOs:
Protein Pacing with Plant-Based Food Options

Specific Food	Grams of Protein per cup	Grams of Fat per cup	Grams of Carbohydrate per cup
Beans, cooked			
Adzuki	17	0	57
Black	15	0	20
Cannellini	17	0	18
Garbanzo	18	.5	46
Navy	15	0	28
Kidney	16	1.5	37.1
Pinto	15	1.9	30
Peas, cooked			
Split peas	16	.8	41
Lentils	18	.9	40

Black-eyed peas	14	1	36
Soy			
Edamame	17	5	26
Soy "nuts"	34	12	16
Tofu (firm)	10	5.9	2.3
Tempeh	18.5 (per 100g)	10.8 (per 100g)	9.4 (per 100g)
Seitan	21 (per 100g)	4.1 (per 100g)	9.9 (per 100g)
Nuts			
Macadamia	12	92	12
Pistachio	12	26	16
Walnut	12	52	11
Almond	30	71	31
Cashew	18	44	30
Pecan	10	78	15
Peanut	38	72	23.5
Seeds			
Pumpkin (pepitas)	48	78.4	17.6
Sunflower	29	72	28
Flax	30.7	71	48
Chia	24.1	44	60

Vegan and Vegetarian Proteins

◊ Beans: adzuki, black, cannellini, garbanzo, navy, kidney, pinto, soybeans, edamame (eat 8–12 oz.)

◊ Peas: split peas, lentils, black-eyed peas (eat 8–12 oz.)

◊ Tofu, tempeh, and seitan (eat 5–7 oz.)

◊ Nuts: macadamia, pistachio, walnut, almond, pecan, peanut, cashew (eat 3.5 oz. unsalted and dry-roasted). Some nuts, such as cashews and peanuts, can also be significant sources of carbohydrate

◊ Seeds: pumpkin (pepitas), sunflower, flax, chia (3.5 oz. unsalted and dry-roasted)

Animal Proteins (Please refer to my cookbook for a more detailed list)

◇ Fish: haddock, cod, scrod, halibut, catfish, crawfish, flounder, herring, perch, sole, trout, clam, tuna, salmon, mackerel, sardines, anchovies, snapper, mahi mahi, shellfish (eat 3.5 oz.)

◇ Eggs: cooked egg whites (eat four egg whites), hardboiled (eat three eggs), scrambled (eat three eggs), egg substitute (eat 5–7 oz.)

◇ Yogurt: Greek yogurt, plain, unsweetened (eat 8 oz.); Greek yogurt, plain, 2% (eat 8.5 oz.); kefir, plain, low-fat (eat 14 oz.); regular yogurt, non/low-fat, plain: (eat 16 oz.)

◇ Cottage cheese: Non-fat cottage cheese (eat 5.5 oz.), 1% low-fat cottage cheese (eat 6 oz.), 2% cottage cheese (eat 8 oz.), 4% cottage cheese (eat 7 oz.)

◇ Milk: whole, preferably from grass-fed cows (drink 20 oz.)

◇ Meat: grass-fed beef, sirloin, or buffalo (eat 3.5 oz.); organic chicken breast (eat 2.5 oz.); chicken, dark meat (eat 2.5 oz.); sliced turkey or ham, try to avoid cold cuts high in sodium or with added sugars (eat 3.5 oz.); ground turkey (eat 3 oz.); turkey breast (2.5 oz.); turkey dark meat (2.5 oz.); pork chop (eat 3 oz.); pork tenderloin (eat 3 oz.).

Don't forget to add your supplements:

Whey Protein

Pea Protein

Legume (Fava, mung, bean) Protein

Brown Rice Protein

Hemp Protein

Bone Broth Protein

Collagen Protein

Get Your Fats:

◇ **Saturated:** Grass-fed butter and clarified butter (ghee); grass-fed beef tallow; duck Fat; full-fat yogurt

◇ **Monounsaturated:** Cold-pressed organic EVOO, avocados, macadamia nuts, almonds, cashews, pistachios

◇ **Polyunsaturated:** Omega-6s and omega-3s from krill oil/sardines, wild-caught salmon; small fish, not farmed, not grain or factory food fed.

◊ **Get Your Carbs:** To maximize nutrient intake per calorie and minimize "empty" carbs that are easily transformed into glucose (fat forming at high levels), the majority of your carbohydrates should come in the form of resistant starches that I described earlier—vegetables and some high-nutrient fruits and berries.

◊ Portion: Eat vegetables with three or more of your "four to six daily mini-meals." Green leafy vegetables can be eaten in abundance, but steam them once they exceed a fist-sized portion.

◊ **Grains in Moderation**: Quinoa, barley, steel-cut oats, wild/brown rice, spelt, resistant starches (Feel free to refer back to my discussion of "Wonder Carbs" in chapter 7 and my cookbook to help guide you through your choices.)

◊ **Vegetables**: Broccoli, kale, escarole, chicory, swiss chard, spinach, collard greens, beet greens, mesculin (can often be a greens salad mix), summer and fall squashes (pumpkin, acorn, butternut), beets, carrots, tomatoes, avocado.

◊ **Fruits in moderation**: Pomegranate, bananas, melons, peaches, mango, oranges, grapefruit, pineapple, kiwi, apples, pears, nectarines, plums

◊ **Berries**: Blueberries, blackberries, acai berries, raspberries, boysenberries, strawberries, cranberries

Grab and Go Options:

If you want to start working your way toward this Protein Pacing style of eating right now—before you even make a trip to the store—I've made this list of fifteen snack and mini-meal options that can be eaten right out of your crisper or pantry. These are good grab-and-go options for travel or during the work day. I make sure I have plenty of these ingredients on hand at all times so I can satisfy any cravings that strike, be it for salty foods or sweet ones.

15 Protein Pacing snacks you can eat right now:

◊ a banana and a hand full of almonds.

◊ a couple of hard-boiled eggs.

◊ a cup of full fat cottage cheese with avocado, sprouts, some nuts or blueberries.

◊ a glass or two of 10 grams of protein unsweetened almond, hemp, or coconut milk with high-fiber whole grain crackers, veggies and nut butter.

◊ a cup of unsweetened full-fat Greek yogurt (preferably from entirely grass-fed cows) with fresh fruit.

◊ whole grain rice cakes with nut or seed butter and sliced fruit with a glass of milk (dairy, almond, coconut, cashew). Remember that dairy milk has roughly 12 g of lactose (milk sugar) per cup. Other milks may prove just as satisfying without the empty carbohydrates.

◊ homemade hummus with veggies.

◊ mixed greens and a can of tuna in water. (If you can find it, tuna in extra virgin olive oil is also a delicious quick meal. Beware of inflammatory vegetable oils, such as canola and soybean oil).

◊ pita wrap with chicken, turkey, or fish and fresh veggies.

◊ a berry smoothie with a scoop of pea, fava, mung, legume, hemp, or undenatured whey protein.

◊ apple slices with natural (preferably organic) peanut butter (Again, look out for added vegetable oils, particularly hydrogenated oils, which are used to extend shelf life and maintain a thick consistency).

◊ handful of assorted nuts and dried fruit (Do your best to avoid dried fruit with added sugar. If you let your taste buds adjust, you will find that unsweetened dried fruit is packed with condensed fruit sugars).

◊ 1 cup of canned or cooked beans (lentils, black/kidney beans, chickpeas, etc.) with rice or quinoa.

◊ homemade turkey meatball pita wrap.

◊ 10 oz. of (unsweetened or lightly sweetened, grass-fed) kefir with almonds or walnuts.

◊ protein powders or bars (homemade or store bought—see my approved list of bars).

PRISE MEAL TIMING CHART:

On these two pages, you will find the meal timing and fitness training schedule that fits your lifestyle. Just simply pick what time of day works best for you to fit in your exercise, and I will help you nourish your body to maximize your results… R-I-S-E UP!

Protein Pacing and Fitness Training Meal Timing Schedule for Resistance (R) and Intervals (I)

Time of Day	Morning Exercise (My Top Pick)	Lunchtime Exercise	After Work Exercise	Evening Exercise (My Last Pick)
6:00AM	WAKE-UP TIME!			
6:15AM	Morning Muscle Maximizer (MMM)	Morning Muscle Maximizer (MMM)	Morning Muscle Maximizer (MMM)	Morning Muscle Maximizer (MMM)
6:30AM	R: 1 hour or I: 30 minutes			
9:30AM	Morning Snack (Optional)	Morning Snack (Optional)	Morning Snack (Optional)	Morning Snack (Optional)
NOON		R: 1 hour or I: 30 minutes		
12:30PM	Lunch		Lunch	Lunch
1:00PM		Lunch		
3:30PM	Afternoon Snack (Optional)		Afternoon Snack (Optional)	Afternoon Snack (Optional)
4:00PM		Afternoon Snack (Optional)		
5:00PM			R: 1 hour or I: 30 minutes	
6:30PM	Dinner		Dinner	Dinner
7:00PM		Dinner		
9:30PM	Bedtime Bellyfat Burner (BBB)		Bedtime Bellyfat Burner (BBB)	R: 1 hour or I: 30 minutes
10:00PM		Bedtime Bellyfat Burner (BBB)		Bedtime Bellyfat Burner (BBB)
10:30PM	BEDTIME...			

Protein Pacing and Fitness Training Meal Timing
Schedule for Stretching (S) and Endurance (E)

Time of Day	Morning Exercise (My Top Pick)	Lunchtime Exercise	After Work Exercise	Evening Exercise (My Last Pick)
6:00AM	WAKE-UP TIME!			
6:15AM	S: 1 hour or E: 1-2 hours	Morning Muscle Maximizer (MMM)	Morning Muscle Maximizer (MMM)	Morning Muscle Maximizer (MMM)
8:00AM	Morning Muscle Maximizer (MMM)			
9:30AM		Morning Snack	Morning Snack	Morning Snack
11:00AM	Morning Snack			
NOON		S: 1 hour or E: 1-2 hours		
12:30PM			Lunch	Lunch
1:30PM		Lunch		
2:00PM	Lunch			
3:30PM			Afternoon Snack	Afternoon Snack
5:00PM	Afternoon Snack	Afternoon Snack	S: 1 hour or E: 1-2 hours	
6:30PM			Dinner	Dinner
8:00PM	Dinner	Dinner		S: 1 hour or E: 1-2 hours
9:30PM			Bedtime Bellyfat Burner (BBB)	
10:00PM	Bedtime Bellyfat Burner (BBB)	Bedtime Bellyfat Burner (BBB)		Bedtime Bellyfat Burner (BBB)
10:30PM	BEDTIME...			

Eating Plus Exercise

Study after study shows that eating the right foods at the right time can actually make you less hungry, that people who work out the right way tend to eat less afterward than those who stay on the couch or who exercise the wrong way. But if you find the opposite to be true—that you want to scarf down pretty much anything in sight after exercise—you're not alone. Many people who begin to exercise also increase food intake. This can sabotage your best diet and healthy eating efforts. If you find yourself wanting to do this, ask yourself why. If you didn't eat a mini protein-packed meal before exercise, chances are you will feel famished when you're done. If you went to an intense cycling class, you may be telling yourself that you "deserve" to take in a few hundred extra calories after all the ones you just burned off. Or if all you do is endurance/aerobic exercise every day hour after hour your hunger cues will scream for food, and lots of it, all the time! Exercise is not a free pass to eat freely and without consequence. If you find this starting to happen, ease off on your exercise for a week until you really get the eating routine down. Once your body and brain know you're taking in more than enough food to fuel your day, add exercise back in. But make sure it's the right exercise, the PRISE Protocol, not just any exercise.

Each time you exercise is an opportunity to build a little more muscle (or a lot, if you're Protein Pacing and **R**esistance strength training with PRISE). Adding more muscle to your frame is one easy way to burn more calories all day long. Studies have shown that adding more muscle can help your body burn hundreds of extra calories a day, especially fat calories. That means you'll be burning more calories every single day—even the days you take off from exercise. Best of all, the more fit you are, the more your lean muscle prefers to get energy from your body fat over any other fuel source.

There's more. Exercise is a proven antidote for stress and anxiety. If you're feeling stressed about work or your home life, you may find you want to sneak in more cookies and chips. (Emotional eating is rarely about overindulging because you're just so happy!) By managing these feelings in healthier ways—through my Stretching and Endurance exercise—you'll save yourself all those extra unwanted calories while tapping into your fat stores for fuel. It's a win-win.

Finally, committing to an exercise routine makes it easier to stick to an eating plan. There's a lot of science to back this up, but you may have noticed it on your own too. When you're able to accomplish one goal, it makes the other ones seem even more within reach. If you start your day with a brisk walk around the neighborhood, you may be less likely to reach for a pastry for breakfast. If you sign up for a fitness class after work, you may be more mindful throughout the day about putting foods into your belly that will fuel you. If you do decide to splurge on the occasional ice cream or candy bar, you'll know exactly how to zap it away—with exercise. This is the synchronicity of using true nourishment with proper amounts of smart exercise to attain optimal health! Please take it from me; I've developed my PRISE Protocol to help you take the road less traveled to optimal health and peak performance because I've done the research for you! One additional point I want leave you with is, I have some exciting new research I will be sharing with all of you very soon on the effects of my Protein Pacing and PRISE Protocol on enhancing your mood – stay tuned!

Thomas Edison could not have been more accurate when he stated, "The doctor of the future will no longer treat the human frame with drugs, but rather will cure and prevent disease with nutrition and food." It's time for us to step into and embrace this future!

15

Sleep or Meditation? Choose Both!

Sleep is that golden chain that ties health and our bodies together.
—Thomas Dekker

Did you ever read the quote by Ernest Hemingway: "I love sleep. My life has the tendency to fall apart when I'm awake, you know?" I am sure we can all relate to that some days! But the truth is we need our sleep, and too many people short-change the quantity (length) and quality of it. I routinely speak to audiences of all sizes, ages, and health statuses across the country on a variety of health, wellness, and fitness topics. Every time I provide the recommended number of hours of sleep, I'm struck by the number of sighs, moans, and even chuckles I hear from the audience due to their shortcoming of meeting the required goal of seven to eight hours per night for adults and nine-plus hours for those under eighteen years old.

In reality, most people fall well-below these sleep recommendations, and for those close to meeting the recommendation, the quality (depth) of their sleep is often lacking. Research studies consistently show that poor sleep quantity and quality are related to increased risk of health conditions, such as heart disease, high blood pressure, diabetes, obesity, depression, and stress, as well as decreased brain function (cognition).[80,81]. Sleep loss is also related to increased drug use among adolescents.[82]

---

80   Jean-Philippe Chaput et al., "Seven to Eight Hours of Sleep a Night Is Associated with a Lower Prevalence of the Metabolic Syndrome and Reduced Overall Cardiometabolic Risk in Adults," PLOS ONE. Accessed March 11, 2018. http://journals.plos.org/plosone/article?id=10.1371%2Fjournal.pone.0072832.

81   J. P. Chaput et al., "Longer sleep duration associates with lower adiposity gain in adult short sleepers," *Nature News*, June 07, 2011. Accessed March 1, 2018. http://www.nature.com/articles/ijo2011110.

82   Sara C. Mednick, Nicholas A. Christakis, and James H. Fowler, "The Spread of Sleep Loss Influences Drug Use in Adolescent Social Networks," PLOS ONE. Accessed March 1, 2018. http://journals.plos.org/plosone/article?id=10.1371%2Fjournal.pone.0009775.

Lifestyle choices such as good nutrition, exercise, and mind-body techniques (mindfulness, meditation, etc.) have a powerful impact on improving both sleep quality and quantity.

Here are some of these strategies...

Nutrition and Sleep

Trim the fat and sugar: In the _Journal of Clinical Sleep Medicine_,[83] a group of researchers demonstrated that diets containing lower fiber and higher saturated fat and sugar are linked with lighter, less restorative sleep that included a longer time to fall asleep and more arousals (periods of awakening). The study showed that slow wave sleep, which is the deepest, most restful sleep, and the time needed to fall asleep were the most negatively impacted by a poor diet. So... reducing fat and sugar intake close to bedtime is a "no-brainer." Instead, I strongly recommend a high-fiber and lean protein meal or snack one to two hours prior to your bedtime (BBB smoothie is ideal) to maximize sleep duration and depth.

Bean me up!: In a similar study called "Beans Improve Sleep,"[84] a group of scientists analyzed the diets and sleep patterns of more than a thousand adults. Their findings revealed that, among the study population, the prevalence of adequate quantity and quality of sleep was not good, 13% and 56%, respectively. But the biggest takeaway was that optimal sleep duration and depth (quality) was greatest among those individuals with the highest intake of foods containing the plant chemicals known as isoflavones (daidzein genistein) found in soybeans, chickpeas, and other legumes. My other top nutrition choices to aid sleep include 4–8 oz. of tart cherry juice, 4–7 oz. of pumpkin seeds, 200 mg of magnesium citrate, 1-5 mg of melatonin, and avoid all caffeine from noon on.

Exercise, Environment, and Sleep

Staying physically active is a natural sleeping aid as well, but limit performing vigorous exercise within one to two hours of going to bed at night.

The virtues of napping have been around for a long time, and for good reason, especially following a sleep-deprived night. If you find yourself dozing off

---

83 "Fiber and Saturated Fat Are Associated with Sleep Arousals and Slow Wave," National Center for Biotechnology Information, Accessed March 3, 2018. https://www.ncbi.nlm.nih.gov/pubmed.

84 Yufei Cui et al., "Relationship between daily isoflavone intake and sleep in Japanese adults: a cross-sectional study," _Nutrition Journal_, December 29, 2015. Accessed March 3, 2018. https://nutritionj. biomedcentral.com/articles/10.1186/s12937-015-0117-x.

at your desk at work, steal away a short ten- to twenty-minute nap, and chances are you will feel refreshed, mentally sharp, and ready to move your body. As one article states, "A Nap Is Smart."[85]

Here are a few additional strategies to a better night's sleep:

◊ Keep a routine, especially wake-up time: Having a consistent bedtime schedule is good for everyone, but a regular rise time in the morning is even more important for healthy sleeping.

◊ Hibernate like a bear and create your own cave: A dark, cool (58–64°F) room is best for deep sleep, just like hibernating animals. Try a sleeping mask if the room has too much natural light.

◊ Avoid the caffeine buzz after breakfast: Limit caffeine-containing foods/drinks after the morning meal.

◊ Unplug!: Emerging research is showing that the backlight from cell phones and other mobile devices (e-readers, laptops, etc.) remain illuminated inside the brain hours after you turn them off and affect your sleep quality and mood.[86] So, unplug at least two hours before you hit the pillow.

◊ Body visit: Obviously, this is my go-to and hope you make it yours (see next section).

◊ Fine tuning your sleep: Avoid intense exercise in the evening; if you drink alcohol, do so in moderation; eat your dinner meal slowly; and minimize spicy foods and gassy foods.

And don't ever underestimate the value of just breathing. Deep-breathing techniques have existed and used by yogis and others through the centuries, and to this date we are still learning about all the hidden value in something as simple as paying attention to your breathing. Shallow breathing is problematic, and for some reason our bodies seem to resort to this when we are under stress or nervous. If we simply paid attention and took deep breaths, we could help ourselves tremendously. Also, when we breathe deeply in meditation or

---

85 J. Waterhouse et al., "The role of a short post-lunch nap in improving cognitive, motor, and sprint performance in participants with partial sleep deprivation.," *Journal of Sports Sciences*, December 2007. Accessed March 15, 2018. https://www.ncbi.nlm.nih.gov/pubmed/17852691.

86 Charles R. Elder et al., *International Journal of Obesity* (2005), January 2012. Accessed March 20, 2018. https://www.ncbi.nlm.nih.gov/pmc/articles/PMC3136584.

throughout the day, we can help accelerate metabolism because, quite simply, we are allowing more oxygen into the bloodstream. To be clear, the type of breathing I am talking about is inhaling deeply but also *exhaling* deeply! Don't hold your breath whether in exercise or in yoga; it is better when you breathe in a deep and rhythmic manner. It actually helps your digestion to burn fat as fuel, and without enough oxygen, the food just can't metabolize. Additionally, the deep-breathing portion brings oxygen in, while the exhale of carbon dioxide helps your body get rid of noxious gases and toxins.

One of my favorite breathing exercises I highly recommend any time during the day whether at rest or in preparing for exercise is diaphragmatic or belly breathing, sometimes called mindfulness breathing. Here how it works:

◊ Either close your eyes or gaze gently five to seven feet in front of you.
◊ Begin by inhaling slowly using a five-second count.
◊ Hold your breath for three seconds.
◊ Exhale to a count of seven.

Repeat until you feel relaxed and in a new state of peacefulness and harmony. As you become more and more comfortable with this technique, extend the time for each phase until you are closer to a seven-second inhale, five-second hold, and nine- to ten-second exhale.

Before I end this section, I want to share just a little about the importance of meditation. Initially, I was reluctant to share this with all of you, but for the better part of those twelve years where my wife and I were completely "maxed" out on life, I suffered terribly from panic disorder. It became so overwhelming at times I couldn't leave the house for days and I was in and out of doctors' offices daily for weeks on end. Life was rough during this time… thankfully, with the help of my wife and family and a continual dose of mind-body training (and prayer), I was able to eventually pull myself out of this abyss. I have two specific "Emotional Nourishment" life-saving techniques I want to share with you. I call them the Body Visit and Mindfulness Awareness Meditation (MAM) because they provide the emotional nourishment we need to keep us in balance and harmony, as well as moving and motivated. These bring all the forms of nourishment together to harmonize our bodies and bring us into fully integrated humans of spirit, mind, and body. You can attain emotional/spiritual fulfillment in several ways. In certain cases, I encourage people to engage in either of these two forms while they are doing other types of PRISE activities, such as stretching or endurance exercises.

Body Visit:

The most common experience of the Body Visit nourishment is through meditation or prayer. There are many different forms of meditation, but my favorite is fairly straightforward. A simplified version of this was initially taught to me by my oldest brother, John, at a time when I was struggling to find emotional fulfilment in my own life. You can choose to do the Body Visit in one of three body positions: seated in a chair with feet on floor, back straight, and arms relaxing gently by your side with your hands resting on your lap; seated in cross-legged position on the floor with a comfortable cushion beneath you with your arms resting on your thighs and palms facing the sky; or lying on your back in the "savasana" position with your legs spread apart, your feet flopping to the side with the flesh of your gluteals pulled out from under you so the lower part of your spine is resting on the floor, your arms extended away from your body, and your palms turned up to the sky with your shoulders relaxed away from your ears.

Once in the position chosen, start by performing several deep abdominal breaths referred to as "diaphragmatic breathing" or "belly breathing" (also called *pranayama*) in yoga, whereby you inhale your breath down into the lowest part of the lungs, causing the abdomen (belly) to rise and fall on inhalation and exhalation. In fact, research shows this type of breathing reduces oxidative stress and increases antioxidant defense status in athletes.[87] Following three deep abdominal breaths, perform two more, but this time, as you inhale, close your eyelids and slowly roll your eyes counterclockwise (actually imagine turning back the clock of time!) by starting with your eyes staring downward and then slowly rolling counterclockwise until you are staring skyward but keeping your eyes closed the entire time. Try to keep your inhalation to five seconds. When you reach the end of inhalation, hold for three seconds with your eyes looking upward. Start your exhalation and continue rolling your eyes in the same counterclockwise direction, arriving back

87   Daniele Martarelli et al., Evidence-based Complementary and Alternative Medicine: eCAM, 2011. Accessed March 20, 2018. https://www.ncbi.nlm.nih.gov/pmc/articles/PMC3139518/.

to where you started with your eyes gently gazing downward. The exhalation should be seven seconds. Perform this two times and, with practice, try pausing in between your inhalation and exhalation for four seconds. With each breath, feel the new air reaching all the way down to your toes and fingertips. Begin to release any tension you are feeling throughout your body.

Continue to breathe in a relaxed, deep, and consistent manner as you feel your body letting go of all tension with each exhalation. During each inhalation feel fresh, new, relaxing, and revitalizing air circulating throughout your body. Once you feel connected to your breath, move on to another common form of meditation referred to as contraction-relaxation meditation. Starting with your forehead, eyes, cheeks, lips, and other muscles of your face, along with your neck muscles, forcefully contract each of them by contracting/tensing all of them for two to four seconds, then let them completely relax by having your eyelids fall over your eyes and allowing your mouth to hang open. Feel your ears begin to relax to the ground. Next, tighten all the muscles in your shoulders, upper back, arms, and hands by clenching your fists and shrugging your arms and shoulders up to your ears and hold for two to four seconds, and then exhale and completely relax all of these muscles. Allow your hands to open to the sky and your shoulder blades to sink to the ground. Imagine all the muscles of your arms completely melting down to the ground and becoming very heavy. Continue this same process with the rest of your body, next with the abdomen, hips, thighs, gluteals, legs, calves, and feet until you've contracted and relaxed all the muscles in your body so you are fully aware of how you are feeling.

Once you've completed both the belly breathing and the contraction-relaxation meditation, begin to feel the tension disappear from your forehand, eyes, mouth, cheeks, and neck muscles. Allow your mouth to hang open and the small of your neck begin to soften and sink to the ground. Allow your ears to relax and all the muscles of your face to sink to ground. Next, bring your attention to your shoulders, arms, and hands. Release the tension between your shoulder blades by pulling your shoulders and arms away from your spine so that you have created more space between your shoulder blades. Again, feel your belly rising with each breath in (inhale) and falling with each breath out (exhale). Your exhalation should last longer than your inhalation and provide you with a feeling of deeper relaxation. Finally, feel the muscles of your hips, thighs, calves, and feet begin to relax and sink down away from your bones so they feel heavy and loose. You are now ready to begin your journey into the Body Visit mindfulness awareness meditation.

With your body in a new state of relaxation, allow any thoughts entering your mind to pass by without holding any judgment to them. Imagine each thought as a raindrop hitting your car windshield and the wipers passing over the window clearing them away from your windshield so that none of them stay very long but instead get wiped away with each passing of the wiper blade. Another way to deal with your thoughts is to imagine them scrolling by as a ticker tape passes highlights or news events at the bottom of your TV screen; none of them stay longer than a few seconds. The true value of the Body Visit is it allows us to move from a state of human nature (also known as subconscious) into a state of higher nature or superconscious. This allows us to "drop into" what many refer to as the "flow state," a higher level of living and experiencing life. The flow state allows us to be in a higher nature and live to our full potential with creativity, problem solving, and freedom. One strategy that I've used since I was a young boy is the Guided Body Visit.

Guided Body Visit with Imagery:

For this meditation, it's best to lie flat on your back in the "savasana" pose described above. Once you feel your mind has emptied, begin to transport yourself in your mind to a place that makes you feel completely relaxed and content and in harmony, such as lying on a beautiful beach; on the top of a mountain peak; in the woods in a clearing with treetops overhead; or in a green pasture. Create a picture of you being a part of this ideal, peaceful serene environment where you are completely relaxed and content. With each breath, allow your body to feel and hear the same sensations as you would if you were actually in that place. Using the beach as the example, imagine lying on a soft beach towel on the warm beach sand underneath an umbrella on a beautiful blue sky and bright sunshine day. Feel the warmth of the sand underneath you and the sun shining all around you, the cool, refreshing spritzing salty breeze of the ocean mist as it floats into the air and gently covers your body. Hear the gentle rumble of the ocean waves splashing onto the shore, one after another. If you are in the mountains, woods, or are in a green grass pasture, breathe in the fresh, crisp air and feel it enter your lungs. Look with amazement at all of the vibrant colors and living species that nature has to offer and then observe all of the unique and special sounds of the birds, insects, and other animals as they speak to each other and to you. For consistency, I will use the reference of the imagery of the beach scene moving forward. With each gentle breaking of the waves, your breathing becomes deeper, more relaxed, and your mind brings your body closer to actually being a part of the beach. Begin to snuggle your toes and then your feet beneath the warm soft beach sand. Off in the near distance, feel a sense of complete harmony as the waves softly roll onto shore and then retreat back out into the ocean, and just beyond that you hear the innocent laughter from young children experiencing joy, or the wonderful sounds of the birds singing in harmony with the wind. Bring in the moment, in the same place that brings you total and complete peace and harmony.

The best part of this meditation is that it can be performed at any time of day wherever you can find a quiet place to lie down for five to fifteen minutes. I enjoy practicing it upon waking in the morning to start my day in harmony or following my stretching exercise routine or at the end of a busy/hectic day to unwind. However, when I want to positively influence my physical performance whether at work, before an important presentation, or at an athletic competition, I will perform my Body Visit along with the Mindfulness Awareness Meditation.

Mindfulness Awareness Meditation

This is, by far, my favorite type of emotional/spiritual nourishment when I'm preparing for a performance of any kind. Once I've completed the basic Body Visit or the Guided Body Visit with imagery, as I lie on my back completely relaxed, I place myself in the same naturalistic environment each time to build consistency, which strengthens the effectiveness of the meditation. I create an image of me walking in a beautiful soft green grass field on a warm sparkling sunny day with weeping willow trees providing occasional overhead shade. I remain captivated by the majestic beauty of the vibrant colors of the rich, dark green grass, the deep blue sky, bright yellow-orange sun, and the exuberant multicolored flowers strewn across the pasture. There is a gentle breeze blowing to keep me cool as I slowly stroll down the green grass pasture. I am dressed in a loose-fitting soft cotton button-down short-sleeved shirt and comfortably fitted soft cotton shorts. On my feet are open sandals that allow my feet to feel the open air and warm sun and the soft touch of the grass beneath my feet. As I slowly walk down the slopes of the grassy field, I come to a circular cement patio with a beautiful water fountain in the middle. The fountain is surrounded by a waist-high brick foundation with marbletop finish. As I approach the fountain, I take in the majestic beauty and notice the reflection of the sun sparkling off each water droplet emanating from the fountain as it spouts water out the top. When I reach the fountain, I place my left hand on the cool marble finish atop the brick wall surrounding the fountain and slowly walk around the fountain starting on the right side and make one complete circle around, and then I turn back and place my right hand on the marble finish and walk back halfway. I then proceed walking down the grassy green pasture enjoying the cornucopia of colors and fresh smells of the grass, trees, flowers, and the warmth of the sun on my body. I arrive at another fountain of similar design as the one before. I follow the same movement pattern of walking completely around once from the right side then turning slowly and walking back halfway around in the opposite direction, again placing my right hand atop the marble surface. I continue with this same pattern of walking down this gently sloping soft bright-green grassy field, passing under the weeping willows that allow the warm sun to peak through the branches while my feet enjoy the softness of the cushioned grass beneath me and the sweet smell of flowers and grass along the way. The number of fountains that I come across is entirely dependent upon the depth of the meditative state I am seeking to obtain. Regardless of how long I stroll in the grass field and the number of fountains I come across, my main focus is on the moment and the sensations I experience along the way. In fact, the longer my stroll and time in this meditative state the more I become attuned to other sounds, sights, smells, and happenings around me in nature, such that my awareness becomes "super-heightened." I begin to notice birds chirping in the trees, the unique colors on the butterflies' wings floating in front of me, and the bees pollinating the flowers along my walk.

Each step brings a greater awareness of my surroundings and things I might not necessarily pay attention to any other time in my waking life. It is both exhilarating and entirely relaxing at the same time to soak up all the beauty of nature while allowing my body to reach a new state of awareness, focus, and relaxation.

This heightened sense of being is an ideal place to allow the final step of meditation to occur. As I pass by the last fountain in the pasture, I allow myself to enter an environment in which I start off as a spectator in the audience watching a person "perform" a perfectly executed performance, whatever it might be.

As I'm sitting observing the performance, without passing any judgment, criticism, or comment, I soon become aware that the person I am observing is me. I sit calmly observing myself perform in an admiring way, passing no judgment either good or bad. I am simply content watching myself perform. The primary reason I sit in content admiration is because my performance is flawless, near perfect in every way. It does not matter if I am in front of 100,000 people in a packed stadium giving a speech or performing one of the many athletic contests I compete in. I am performing effortlessly and completely calm and content; there is no tension in my body or mind anywhere. I am poised, engaging, and in control no matter the circumstance. If I know going into my meditation who my audience or opponent will be, I anticipate this and put them in the appropriate place and even have them challenge me in some way. My response is always precise, correct, and performed with quiet confidence and poise. I observe myself from the position of the spectator or audience for the first couple of minutes but then zoom in close to myself and transition into the view of actually performing the action. Similar to my audience view, I perform now as myself and continue to execute and perform with complete effortlessness, flow, and with ease and poise. My breathing, heart rate, and mind are in harmony and rhythmical despite the gravity of the environment that I am performing. I am completely in harmony with mind, body, and spirit yet fully aware and present in the moment. I call it mind-body-spirit-fullness, and I feel fully integrated as a human being. It's a supreme state of being, one I want to inhabit as often as possible, and I want you to experience this too! The good news for all of you is, with practice, you can achieve this state in as little as five to ten minutes a day.

Peace comes from cultivating the time to find it. It is there waiting for you at all times, *if* you stop long enough to recognize it. If you don't, then you spin yourself into situations and lives that you would really rather not manifest. The human body needs its refreshing and restorative sleep, and the proper emotional nurturance as well. If you can incorporate some of the meditations, what you will find is the use of your time will become so much more efficient, focused, and clear. The newly found energy and intent behind your thoughts and actions will assure that you aren't wasting valuable time with anxiety and negative thinking but will provide you a renewed life to reach your goals. They are the "golden chains" that Thomas Dekker refers to that keep your body/mind strong, healthy, and connected.

16

The Ultimate PRISE
An "App": Your Trusted
24-Hour Coach

PRISE Nutrition, Fitness, and Health App

"How many calories have you eaten today?" "How many steps have you taken today?" The modern world is so very different! If you're one of the millions of people tracking every morsel of food you've eaten using MyfitnessPal or FatSecret or wearing a fitness-tracking device, such as the Fitbit, Jawbone Up, Nike Fuelband, Basis Peak, Garmin Vivofit, the latest Apple Health Watch, or even using a similar app like Google Fit or Moves, the answer is at your fingertips. In fact, you probably know how many calories you've burned too.

An eye-opening statistic stated that there were 90 million wearable nutrition, fitness, and health-monitoring devices sold in 2014, and it has projected the market will grow from $4 billion in 2015 to over $40 billion in 2020![88] So, what makes these nutrition, health, and fitness-tracking devices so popular? For most people, it's the awareness of eating an appropriate number of calories and staying active during the day, especially if you haven't met your "step" or "calorie" goal. To put it simply, they motivate you to remain active and eat the appropriate number of calories, and they do a good job accomplishing this goal.[89]

But these nutrition, fitness, and health self-monitoring devices attempt to do so much more than just record steps and calories. Some measure heart

---

88 Tim Bajarin, "Fitbit: Here's Why Fitness Trackers Are Here to Stay," *Time*. June 24, 2015. Accessed March 3, 2018. http://time.com/3934258/fitness-trackers-fitbit/.
89 David Pogue, "Fitness Trackers Are Everywhere, but Do They Work?" *Scientific American*. January 01, 2015. Accessed March 2, 2018. https://www.scientificamerican.com/article/fitness-trackers-are-everywhere-but-do-they-work/.

rate, blood oxygen level, respiration rate, skin temperature, sweat rate, sleep patterns, etc. and soon they will be capturing vital personal biometrics, such as blood sugar, blood pressure, and blood lipids. A word of caution: because these self-monitoring devices are undergoing such a rapid evolution, a major concern is their ongoing accuracy. Indeed, a recent article in *JAMA* highlights the variability of measurement (accuracy) among these different devices.[90]

As a matter of interest, I've been publishing scientific research studies using data from these technologies and devices (apps, accelerometers) for over a decade, so they're not "new" to me. The ones I use for my scientific research studies have been validated and shown to be fairly accurate. I cannot say the same for the ones currently on the market. In any case, they were originally developed to provide an estimate, not a direct measure of the calories eaten and the calories burned during physical activity, so it's probably not a wise idea to create a "balance sheet" of the calories burned using these devices and the calories you are allowed to eat. This approach will leave you frustrated because you'll be either starving or plump.

In my view, a major limitation of *all* the current self-monitoring nutrition, health, and fitness technologies and tracking devices, whether it's a wearable tracking device or a mobile health app, is their overzealous focus on measuring the "quantity" of each lifestyle metric. Their goal is a *zero-sum game* of quantifying (measuring) the "number" of steps, calories, sleep, heart rate, breaths, beads of sweat, etc. and there is little if any attention to the "quality" (type) of these lifestyle experiences. In support of this, countless well-respected scientists and studies have documented that the *quality* of our lifestyle choices is much more important than the *quantity* of each of these aspects of health.

For example, simply recommending "more" exercise as a public health initiative is considerably less effective than encouraging a balanced routine incorporating a variety of movement experiences, such as resistance, interval, stretching, and endurance exercises as part of my PRISE Protocol. And I have the published research to back this up. Similarly, telling someone to simply "eat less" to lose weight is not very helpful, healthy, or motivating in the long term. Whereas, providing help and guidance with choosing the right type of high-quality, nourishing foods, especially protein using my Protein Pacing plan, is

90   Meredith A. Case, "Accuracy of Devices to Track Physical Activity Data," *JAMA*. February 10, 2015. Accessed March 3, 2018. https://jamanetwork.com/journals/jama/fullarticle/2108876#tab1.

paramount to effective, healthy weight loss and body composition. Recently, I've been interviewed to comment on these nutrition and fitness technologies and tracking devices, and you can watch it at "Dr. Paul on Look TV".[91] My take-home message emphasizes the potential benefit these technologies will provide for workplace wellness to increase productivity, morale, and, most importantly, health. The cost savings will be enormous to employers, employees, and the entire workforce.

Herein lies the next phase of nutrition, health, and fitness technologies (wearables and apps). The industry is primed to develop a combination nutrition/health app and fitness tracking device that emphasizes the *quality* of lifestyle choices above and beyond the quantified self. Fortunately, I've been consulted by the health and wellness and health-care industries to provide a novel approach of personalized nutrition, fitness, and emotional well-being using my PRISE Life App. On the horizon, is full integration with Apple Healthkit and wearable devices to guide users in a fully customized experience that also links their biometrics in real-time with thier health and fitness goals to optimize the PRISE Life experience. The PRISE App offers an individualized navigational tool that guides the user to the appropriate lifestyle choice to either lose weight, increase energy, or improve physical/athletic performance with the primary goal of enhanced health, fitness, and wellness but without *all* the logging!

Ultimately, the PRISE App aims to drastically improve the way we deliver personal self-care, optimal health, and peak performance at a global level. Fortunately, health-care providers (physicians, etc.) and insurers (organizations) are fully onboard with giving more ownership to individuals (employees, patients, etc.) to monitor their own health metrics so they can reduce health-care insurance premiums and medical costs; this way, both sides feel incentivized.

Ideally, if we can get health-care providers and insurers to consistently prescribe and encourage health apps like PRISE, it will benefit everyone by motivating them to begin a healthier lifestyle or enhance the experience of those who already engage in a healthy lifestyle. The PRISE App provides the ultimate user experience because it guides the user on a moment-by-moment basis during the day to choose the most effective lifestyle strategy to enhance health and performance based on a customized personal experience unique to each

---

91   Previously featured: http://www.looktvonline.com/look-at-health-fitness-technology/.

individual. In other words, PRISE self-care in your pocket!

I'm most excited to be able to offer my PRISE App (Apple App Store and Android Play Store) to all of you as a companion tool to this book to create a lifestyle you can stay committed to and experience the best results ever! The PRISE App is the first app of its kind that does not rely on logging your food or exercise but instead is designed to "guide" you to making the next best lifestyle strategy based specifically on your personal profile and goals, so it's a customized and individualized experience. The underlying algorithms are based on my thirty years of research and discovery of Protein Pacing and PRISE to engage the user in a unique, one-of-a-kind experience that is specific to them individually to provide the best results! Essentially, the special sauce/secret formula of PRISE are the algorithms I've developed over decades to give the user an individual experience like no other app on the market. It's like having Dr. Paul and PRISE with you all the time! Make sure you go check it out and join us at and www.paularciero.com, www.proteinpacing.com, and priseprotocol.com.

17

Conclusion

The future depends on what you do today.
—Mahatma Ghandi

I hope that after reading this book you are beginning to understand the reason why I thrive on scientific research and am so very excited to share my discoveries with the world!

I hope I have earned your trust and proven to you that the environment from which I conduct my research, teach my students, coach my athletes, and mentor and guide my clients has been at the core of everything I do. It is this atmosphere that has created a rock-solid foundation for my Protein Pacing and PRISE lifestyle strategies (and PRISE App) to assure that they survive "the test of time" and serve millions more well into the futureKnow that I am the actual scientist (with the help of incredible colleagues and research subjects) who made these discoveries and conducted the research that has now been reviewed worldwide. I am used as the leading authority in nutrition and applied physiology, and I am humbled and honored to be *that* Dr. Paul.

Millions and millions of people are finally understanding how the world has changed even in the last five and a half decades I have been alive. With over thirty of those years dedicated to nutrition and exercise physiology—with the value and importance of Protein Pacing—the value of eating protein at proper times, teaching more about how metabolism works, debunking "diet" myths, sharing the proper way to exercise without overexertion, and letting Mother Nature guide us as to how our bodies should really operate, I hope you can see why my enthusiasm never fades.

I want you to get truly *nourished*, emotionally, as well as physically by understanding the value of good nutrition and proper nourishment. No more "calorie counting" and consuming fake processed food. Self-care is the new health-care, and you must be proactive. By following my protocols, you may live a longer and healthier life. I've tested my PRISE Protocol on super-fit men and women, and they out-perform their non-PRISE counterparts in every measure of physical performance too! This is why this is not a diet, it is not a temporary fix, it is a lifestyle plan that will work the rest of your life. Imagine, finally knowing that you can end the diet roller coaster and settle in for the rest of your life in an excellent, not-too-intense, great-tasting, satiating, never hungry, "non-diet" eating for life program, one that keeps you healthy and does not deprive you.

We, as a society, have to end this deadly cycle of obesity, the rat race of over-stress and immobility, the addiction to alcohol and drugs—prescribed or not—which would diminish if we just felt better and could finally claim the ultimate health and peak performance we all so deserve. There is nothing as important as you, your health, and staying motivated so that you can achieve all the things you have set out in this lifetime. We deserve to remain as healthy as possible well into our 80s, 90s, and above. Maybe we will become the civilization that heeded the truth and can live to be the 120 years we were supposed to live to.

We no longer need to be controlled by bad research, misinformation, or bad strategies for living a healthy life. Whether you are running a marathon, an Olympic athlete, or just a person hoping to feel their best every day, there is now nothing stopping you from not only "keeping your eyes on the prize" but actually getting and staying there. The power of *intention* is with you. That intention can become a movement just as people in the past have been moved when societies and races have been mistreated because of lack of knowledge. We can be the "change agents" together!

Being free from having to diet and exercise to an extreme another day, feeling great, and being able to claim your *essence* and complete your *mission* is something not only worth dreaming about but worth working toward. You will finally achieve this because you feel great, and as a result of healthy eating and true nourishment, you will look great! Remember, eat dirty! Live the way nature intended—without overexertion, dehydration, crazy 500-calorie-a-day diets, injections, steroids, medications, bypass surgeries, sugar-packed meal replacement powders, stimulants, deprivation, overanalyzing, and the list goes on. I have learned so much from *her*, so can you!

Nature has truly been a huge source of personal inspiration. It refreshes me daily with new lessons and then provides me with the drive to motivate and help you succeed. For me, this as well as my diverse life experiences have forged an unquenchable desire to commit my life to serving others by providing the permanent lifestyle strategies changes that I have shared.

I had some rough starts myself, and because of a twelve-year insane schedule, I was forced to find a program that would work for *all* people, at all fitness and weight levels, lacking time in their day! Now, my discoveries can change the world! I can't wait to get out and help others, like you, who are the overstressed working moms; the fathers with too many jobs; the families caring for sick loved ones while trying to stay healthy themselves; the students and athletes driven to be the best while holding down other jobs, and so on!

I can't tell you how much I have even learned on this journey while writing this book! Yes, it has been a journey, but I can even say I have evolved, once again, because of it. I even had my virtue revealed to me during a quantum emergence class and discovered it was "kindness." It's known as the "attraction" virtue that is based on appreciating and accepting everyone and everything for its existence as equals. My main goal in life is to bring people together and promote equality and fellowship. See, I've learned even more about myself, and for better or worse, my motivation to get my protocols and knowledge to everyone in the world is through the roof!

I want you to seriously take a commitment moment, take that champion in you, and walk yourself over to the computer or grab your Smart Phone and check out my sites: www.paularciero.com, www.proteinpacing.com, and www.priseprotocol.com. They have all the added pieces that I could not include in this book. Things like more about my PRISE app. It even has a section that lists all my extensive media coverage of research (magazines, newspaper, television, radio appearances), and all of my peer-reviewed published manuscripts for all of you analytical folks!

I encourage you to go check it out and reach out to me. I am here! Even look through the presentations I have done and find the ones of me on YouTube so that you can get me to come speak to your group. We seriously need to create a grassroots effort to get this message out, and no group is too small. I am even working on a way to get an online ecourse and workbook together to teach others how to be my "PRISE Certified Trainers" so even more people can learn and then teach the PRISE Lifestyle. I have a PRISE Fitness training journal and cookbook coming out as well to keep you on track, so the latest material and updates can always be found at www.paularciero.com, www.proteinpacing. com, and www.priseprotocol.com—take a moment to check out where I will be speaking next and bring your book so that I can sign it for you!

My mission has been focused, using scientific methods and research to back up my theories, and with the incredible insights of what our higher power has taught us. I can't help but want you to learn, you to be heard, to overcome whatever physical or intellectual limitation you may have placed on yourself, because with the proper knowledge and guidance that I am handing to you in this book, I know we can make change. It does take a nation, and we are it! I know how supportive my current followers are, so I can't wait to have you behind this movement as well.

Although our journey may be coming to an end in this book, I have provided you a *roadmap* and a book, a website, and even an app so that I am always with you! How wonderful is this interlinked world? It is only with your help that I can really achieve my goals over the coming years, to continue investigating lifestyle-related strategies of nutrition, exercise, and mind/body techniques to facilitate: 1) physical, cognitive, emotional health, and well-being; 2) prevention of cardiovascular, metabolic, cognitive, disease/risk; and 3) optimize physical and athletic performance in people of all ages and health statuses. I want the rest of my life to be devoted to being your global content expert and spokesperson for optimizing health and performance through lifestyle strategies of nutrition, fitness, and mind/body techniques.

With the information I have shared with you in this book, you will find the motivation to throw away all those crazy temporary diet ideas and overexertion exercise fads, look to nature for the answers, and choose optimal health and peak performance. I know you will!

In the end for all of us, though, it is as Ghandi said: "The future depends on what you do today." Let this be the day for you!

In my deepest gratitude, I am so happy to welcome you not only to the team but to your new "PRISE," the Dr. Paul family.

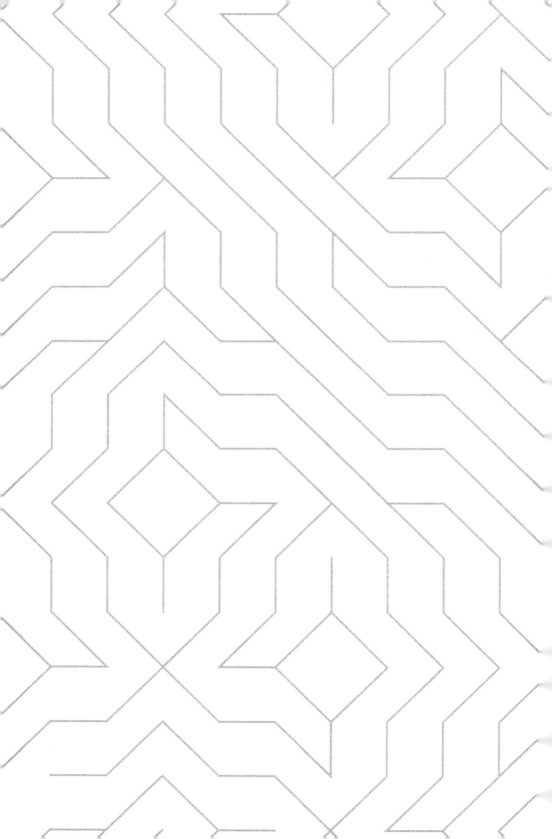

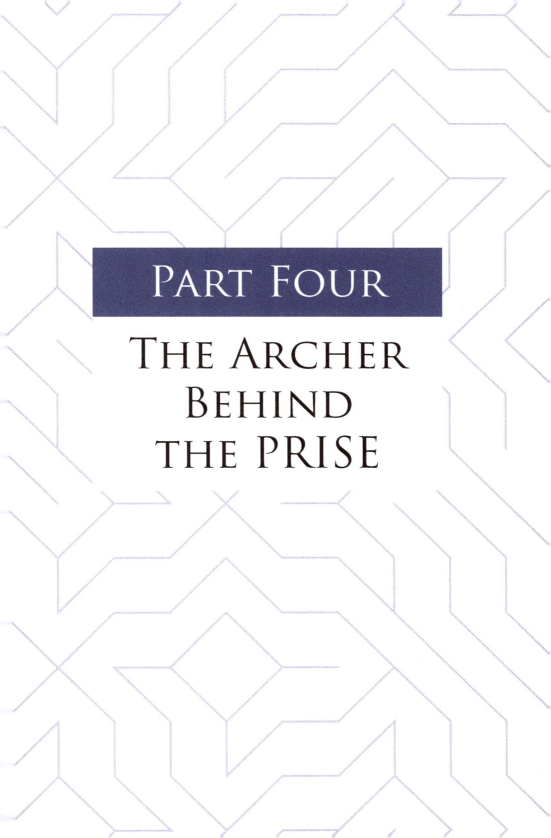

PART FOUR

THE ARCHER
BEHIND
THE PRISE

18

A Mantra from the Author: "Keep Your Eyes on the PRISE!"

It is not the norm for an author to add a section about an inspirational phrase, but to be honest, there is not a lot that is "normal" about this book. Years ago when I created my protocol, this mantra came to me and has always stuck. When people were asked where they thought the phrase, "Keep your eyes on the prize," came from, and what it meant, most thought it was a quote from a champion boxer; some guessed Mohammed Ali. Others felt it was a motivational chant for a sport's team, and only a few were able to source it closer to the truth—and that was mostly because they had probably heard Pete Seeger or Bruce Springsteen utter the words. Few, sadly, got the deeper meaning on how and where the phrase originated. To most, it was a phrase they remembered, and, if they were to guess, it generally meant setting a goal and sticking to it.

In an era where we seem to be just as politically, culturally, and racially charged today as we were half a century ago, technically, even all the way back to the origination of the United States, I thought what better time and way to revive the term and make sure that it's importance was truly understood. (Yes, I took a little creative liberty in the spelling of one word, but I do not want the message or origination of this term lost for a single second.) If you were alive in the 50s and 60s in America, or studied American History, then you know this was the height of racial tensions and the American Civil Rights Movement. To this day, no matter your age, Martin Luther King's "I Have a Dream" speech, followed by his assassination in 1968, brought racial inequality to a head. Brewing long before that, suffrage and separation of black and whites (because that was the term used in those days) created tensions and conflict and separation all over the country, and even on other continents. But somehow, the incredible

gospel songs of the Deep South—that were handed down by word originally—continue to resonate through us to this day. One such song is, "Keep Your
Eyes on the Prize," also known as "Gospel Plow" or "Hold On." Pete Seeger, an
incredible folk singer (who only recently died at age ninety-four) made sure to
introduce the gospel songs to Caucasians and other nationalities as he traveled
the world sharing his *We Shall Overcome* album. His purpose was to not only
keep history and the realization of suffering alive and remembered but share the
power of the words.

The *power* of the words. I don't say that lightly.

There is a power in words, there is a power in intention, and I do not take
any of it lightly. From some research, the true credit of the song is given to:
English Folk Songs from the Southern Appalachians published in 1917, but if you
know your gospel music at all, you know much of it was based on pulling in
strength from God. It was created and sung as rhythmic chants to keep one's
mind and *focus* on something else. In such a time of deep suffering, abuse, pov-
erty, and cruelty, many had to pull on a Higher Power to get through the moment, to survive as a slave one more day. So, for any of you who may have or
have had exposure to Christianity, the Bible, in particular, you will immediately
see the deeper meaning in the words:

Paul and Silas bound in jail
Had no money for to go their bail
Keep your eyes on the prize, hold on

Paul and Silas thought they was lost
Dungeon shook and the chains come off
Keep your eyes on the prize, hold on

Freedom's name is mighty sweet
And soon we're gonna meet
Keep your eyes on the prize, hold on

I got my hand on the gospel plow
Won't take nothing for my journey now
Keep your eyes on the prize, hold on

...

Only chain that a man can stand
Is that chain o' hand on hand
Keep your eyes on the prize, hold on

I'm gonna board that big greyhound
Carry the love from town to town
Keep your eyes on the prize, hold on

...

Now only thing I did was wrong
Stayin' in the wilderness too long
Keep your eyes on the prize, hold on

The only thing we did was right
Was the day we started to fight
Keep your eyes on the prize, hold on

Hold on, hold on
Keep your eyes on the prize, hold on

...

Ain't been to heaven but I been told
Streets up there are paved with gold[92]

Keep your eyes on the prize … hold on! Whether you believe that the Bible is the Word and Truth or you believe that it is a good story (and as you may have heard as a Roman Catholic, *when* you take that wafer and drink that wine in communion it *is* the body and blood of Christ), the deep Southerners held even deeper beliefs, and their God flowed through everything.

This song is no different, but there is a beautiful part of this song that people

---

92   "Pete Seeger, "Keep Your Eyes on the Prize," *Genius*, Pete Seeger Version, accessed February 16, 2018, https://genius.com/Pete-seeger-keep-your-eyes-on-the-prize-lyrics with the chorus removed at ellipses marks.

often miss, and it is the actual story, specifically from Acts 16:19–26 in the Bible, about when good ol' Paul and Silas, both Jews, were marched through town and thrown in jail for *simply not following* the Roman *customs* of the day. They were beaten, starved, stripped naked, and shackled. There was no way out, and nothing was going to save them.

Until…

They started singing hymns that praised God.

Incredible! Envision that you are in the deepest, darkest time of your life, and instead of lashing out in anger, hurt, and fear, you start singing praises to the Creator. That's pretty impressive in my view! I can even share with you that I've been in those moments where there was nothing left to do but cry out for clarity and help.

And if you have never had a chance to truly experience a gospel service in the South, please put it on your bucket list. The incredible energy of groups singing up praise together will change any negativity that is attached to you and might even help move you toward your purpose and release you from your burdens. Sometimes it is what I even feel when I am fortunate enough to stand in front of tens of thousands of people and start to feel the moment of clarity people get when they fully understand and support what I am teaching.

Human energy has power.

So, what happened to Paul and Silas? Just like those hymns where the music wafted through the cotton fields as slaves worked during the day, all the way to the churches on Sunday, the two men's cries were heard. Suddenly, for some unexplained reason, at the very time they sang out, the earth shook, an earthquake took down the entire building, the shackles broke loose, and *all* the prisoners were freed.

That's a Higher Power at work!

I'm not asking anyone to subscribe to a certain religion or belief, but I am asking you to realize that so much of our destiny can be brought into the light by breaking down the wall of lies that we have been told, and I assure you today it feels like the Berlin Wall. My mission has been focused, using scientific methods and research to back up my theories, and with the incredible insights of what our Higher Power has taught us, I can't help but want you to learn, *you* to be heard, and to overcome whatever physical or intellectual limitation you may have placed on yourself, because with the proper knowledge and guidance that I am handing to you in this book, I know we can make change.

Despite the fact—one I am painfully aware of—that I am only a regular scientist guy...I'm not a prophet. I'm a father, husband, brother, son, friend, a coach, a teacher, but something still resonates deeper in me with this phrase. The idea that shackles or limitations can be removed to see the truth and know deep in my soul that I am going to be a major resource, a tiny, human impetus to change—to stop the population from these crazy diet and exercise routines and choose a healthier lifestyle for optimal health and peak performance—then I promise you, I will stay focused and remain committed to you. For *me*, your success *is* the prize. For *me*, I have my *eyes* and heart on you!

For *you*, I have only a few things to ask, as the good song says, help me, help you, "Keep Your Eyes on the PRISE!" Hold on, hold on, because I have a scientifically proven roadmap to take you on. "Freedom's name is mighty sweet," don't you agree? Being free from having to diet and exercise to an extreme another day, feeling great, and being able to claim your *essence* and complete your *mission* is something, because you feeling and looking great is not only worth dreaming about but worth working toward!

I look forward to our journey together, and please know how deeply humbled I am by your support.

Dr. Paul

19

Dr. Arciero (The Archer): Personally Speaking

To this day, it still makes my heart sink when I realize how easy it is for people to look at others and judge; when the truth is, if you heard the stories behind any person's journey, you would most likely hear about some devastating times where people were at their worst, hitting barriers that seemed utterly impossible to rise above. Rest assured, although it might not seem like it now, we all encounter these hard times along the way to finding our true selves or even our "callings." I am no stranger to struggle, and in all honesty, I have had some hard lessons and bumps along the road too. Just like most, or all, of you.

Have they made me stronger?

Have they made me who I am today?

Of course, but they were deeply painful and I will fully disclose my life to all of you.. After all, it may look like I have it all together this moment, but it hasn't always been so easy.

Here's my story.

It is exactly as I shared in the very beginning of this book. I was a terrible student in school from the start. Teachers and administrators asked my parents to hold me back in the first grade and then again in the fifth grade. To make matters worse, my teacher (in the first grade) actually taught me to spell my last name wrong! Not a very good start to life. And the fact that the "higher ups" decided to place me in the slower-moving classes all through elementary, middle, and high school didn't help me feel very confident about any learning experiences.

Fortunately, fate intervened these blows and several early transformative experiences were made available and became vital to keeping me engaged with life. First, my mother, for whatever reason, chose me among her seven children to accompany her to tend our two small 10'X10' plots at the local community garden in the center of downtown near the train tracks and broken down railway station. It was there, beginning in the sunny afternoons of spring, through the hot and muggy days of summer, and ending with the cool brisk days of fall where I would spend hours gardening, just me and my mom. In the most basic sense, this life experience of gardening with my mom at an early age taught me the incredibly important life lesson of nourishing our bodies with the highest-quality food. I also learned why we all need to "get dirty" to eat healthy.

Although I didn't realize it at the time (I was only eight or nine when I started), my mom was developing my appreciation of growing your own food source from the earth's soil and how this is ultimately one of the greatest sources of nourishment to keep our bodies healthy and functioning at the highest level. But in a more philosophical sense, this experience of nurturing a living organism through its life cycle—beginning with the tiny little seed and how to give it just the right amount of water, sun, soil, and protection to support its growth and crop yield—held much more significance. Ultimately, this was the impetus for me choosing the career as a nutrition and exercise scientist with the sole mission of helping others live a lifetime of abundant physical and emotional health as well as optimal performance.

About the same time my mom was developing my appreciation for healthy eating, my dad was supporting my innate need to move my body and be physical. Because I was not a good student, by default, I started to participate in all kinds of movement experiences. I remember being introduced to a trampoline and a climbing rope in gym class, and I immediately started to push my limits while jumping on the trampoline by doing flips and twists. Apparently, I caught the eye of the gym teacher and was invited to show my skill during an evening elementary talent show and tell. During recess, me and my friends would continue with the same flips and twists as I launched myself through the air and let go of the swing, landing in the sand below. I experimented with all sorts of sports and activities, but the two that rose to the top were ice hockey (grew up in New England) and tennis. My early childhood memories of playing youth hockey included my dad gently pulling on my toes under my bed covers at 5:00 a.m. on Saturday morning to get me to 6:00 a.m. outdoor hockey practice in below freezing temperatures; it was called training, but at times felt like cruelty!

But my dad was always smiling and supportive on all those cold mornings and weekend-long tournaments in the wintry cold northeast.

Through high school, my tennis game became increasingly more and more competitive, enough to earn me a scholarship to play in college, despite graduating high school in the lower quartile of approximately 375 students. The defining feature of my early athletic experiences was my dad (and mom) always being there for me and supporting me unconditionally and without criticism or comment, just simply being there for me. I cherish the times we spent together on my journey as an athlete because he (along with my mom) was instrumental in building my self-confidence and self-worth through physical movement and gave me a lifelong appreciation and love of physical movement and my body in motion.

Lastly and perhaps most impactful of my early life experiences, my paternal grandmother and maternal grandfather had a special fondness for me among my six siblings and many other grandchildren who needed their love. I've added photos at the end of this chapter to share some incredible memories and a tiny glimpse into my life.

I would also write letters back and forth regularly with my grandmother, "Grandma Deedie," and they have always touched me deeply. I actually still have some of those letters and show them in my PowerPoint slide presentation when I speak. I can't believe the emotion it still invokes in me every time I look at it or read it. See for yourself. I've added it at the end of this chapter for you to enjoy!

Then there was my grandfather, "Grandpa," who would often whisk me away, just the two of us. These experiences including jumping in his car and going to the local park to play marbles and pitch coins, having him perform magic tricks of pulling quarters or dollar bills from behind my ear, or simply going out for an early morning breakfast at the local diner. Examples of those experiences may seem ordinary, but to me they were totally transformative and left me with a deep feeling of belonging and being loved unconditionally.

Most special for me was my two grandparents believed in me when I didn't believe in myself. Their unwavering love of me kept me in the game of life when I was feeling down and out. Please know, I was blessed to grow up in a loving and nurturing family with loving parents, siblings, grandparents, and relatives, but there were times when life was pretty hectic and chaotic in our house (nine people living in a modest-sized home), and it was easy to get lost in the shuffle. There were even times I would retreat to the car in our driveway to find some peace and quiet to attempt to do my homework back when I was in middle school. Now that alone speaks for the fact that I needed to find some space!

It was the special bonds I developed with my mom, dad, and grandparents that became the core principles of how and why I live my life today. In fact, the love I developed for my parents and grandparents as a child was deep and meaningful and continues to this day. When my grandparents, and eventually my dad's, health began to fail during my teenage years, it broke me, so much so that I dedicated myself to pursue a life (and a career) helping them, and others, live healthier. Their failing health became my life focus, which soon became my life mission and purpose.

But along the way I had my demons surging, and I was starting to fight myself on everything. The quickest way to describe it was that all of a sudden, the false foundations my psyche (mostly that I could only be good if I was the best in a sport) had been standing on all those years came crumbling down, and I simply could not wrap myself around studies or sports and follow through. The net result: I dropped out of college. Yes, you read those words correctly. I was so lost. I was emotional and uncommitted and confused and could not pull it together.

At the same time, I happened to be fortunate enough to have an older brother who was also an accomplished tennis player having just graduated from college as an All-American. It is because of him and this next experience that I can actually pinpoint the exact day, time, and location of my epiphany to dedicate my life to helping others live a life of optimal health and peak performance.

So, I had recently dropped out of college during my sophomore year with a tennis scholarship on the line. My academic demons/weaknesses/failures came back to haunt me, and I started spending too much time on the tennis court instead of the classroom. At the same time, my older brother, and mentor, John, had recently graduated from college, as I said, this "All-American Tennis Player" and decided to compete on the European Satellite tennis tour. So, as a nineteen-year-old college dropout I decided to join him.

About seven weeks into our tennis tour experience I hit rock bottom and had barely won even a match. Then this was the moment the universe stepped in, despite myself.

At the tournament site in St. Girons, France, there was a beautifully serene flowing brook tucked away behind the tennis courts. Before the tournament started, I somehow found myself sitting there beside the brook, mesmerized by the sound of the water gently flowing over the rocks and the glitter of sunshine peeking through the treetops overhead. I remember lying down and going into what I now believe to be a state of mindful awareness meditation that completely transformed my entire body. The only word that comes to mind is I felt I was in perfect harmony—spirit, mind, and body. But the overwhelming mind-set that captured my attention was I knew right then and there what my life was meant and needed to be … service to others by being a resource of optimal health and peak performance. That *single* defining moment changed my life *on the spot* and set me on this journey to bring optimal health and peak performance to others.

Despite the horrendous performance on the tennis court up until this point, this harmony carried over to the tennis court that day, and I won the entire tournament and became a European Tennis Champion! And as I said at the start of this book, the cycle of life threw me yet another one of those dichotomies/paradoxes.

While I should have been gloriously celebrating, a foreign but compelling and immense feeling I had inside me took over, and I was all of sudden "homesick" for my parents, especially my dad. Then, without being able to explain to anyone why, after the most memorable tennis accomplishment in my life up until this time, I made the decision to return home the next week and re-enroll in college.

Several years later, my father would be diagnosed with a very rare form of cancer and pass away at the young age of sixty-one. I was destined and needed to come home. And from this "win" it was the pain of missing family that brought me back to start my next life cycle. My commitment to school, education, getting degrees, research, my scientific mind, the love of nutrition and exercise physiology, putting all the pieces together, and coming up with the discoveries I shared in part 2 now all seem to make sense. These experiences really do form who we are and what we are meant to be. Life, by the struggles and successes, forged an unquenchable desire in me to commit my life to serving others by providing lifestyle strategies for a life of optimal health and peak performance and have landed me here in front of you today.

I must admit that even writing this paragraph now makes me emotional. Very much like when I think of those early days and family, if you have ever attended one of my speeches, you will have seen that my eyes will well up with tears, and I will actually choke up a little bit with emotion when I talk about them and some of my discoveries. Part of that is natural; I'm Italian after all. As I joke, however, the other part as I think about is that sometimes I am just as astounded to be standing here sharing as you may be at learning the material I'm sharing. The fact that I am actually writing this or standing in front of you pouring my heart out touches me because I feel hopeful that it will be the impetus, the strength, that makes you wake up, take action, and make a change in your own life or help someone you love.

And sometimes I'm just hit with an overwhelming sensation of gratitude of, "Holy wow, I'm really here and it's amazing!" Perhaps it's that the older I get as I see my children grow and feel the deep appreciation for the love of my wife and family that I realize how strange it is to have been born into this family at this time with the characteristics I have been granted, both good and bad.

Funny, along the way at some point, I learned about some of my Southern Italian heritage including my name "Arciero," which translated into English means "The Archer" or "The Bowman," and it has become a fun exploration of how there might be something to a name. (As if the Italian first name *Paul* and second name *Joseph* isn't enough!) History, genealogy, and mythology can all have some fascinating revelations as we work to discover who we were born to become.

I do believe that the name and the family you are born into, as well as the life experiences along the way, influence the personality you adopt. I was intrigued about the symbology and heritage behind the archer, especially when I read that an archer is born and driven to hit the mark. They have an internal, unquenchable need to take a specific area of focus and—with incredible forethought, great strength, clarity of attention, the ability to cut out all the other noise, created internally or externally—work repeatedly for many years to get that bow to hit its mark, dead center. Now that I look back at my discoveries, in an odd sense this is exactly what I have done!

For some it may seem easy standing up in front of a huge audience talking about what you do or have done, but it takes feeling well, getting excited time after time, and making sure that you are connecting with the audience at all times, because without that, there is no purpose in standing in front of a huge audience and simply talking away about nothing. How amazing it is that I learned this skill young. Can anyone guess how? Tennis. Of all things. The sport that makes you focus on one ball at all times, keeping pace, and blocking out everything around you with an intensity of focus; that is what leads to winning the ultimate prize—in this case a long and healthy life.

In the end, looking back over my life and at the incredible nurturing from those who saw something in me—something in me that was needed for the rest of the world that I couldn't see myself—and took action whether it was taking me to play in the garden, encourage me by wiggling my toes to get up in unforgiving weather to go play hockey, or those who made sure that they told me how special I was *exactly* as I was, when I couldn't see it myself. That is powerful. That is humbling and shows me how little control we have over the ages and stages of our lives, as I mentioned in the introduction. Even the bad times where I felt humiliated, uninspired, and like I may have blown it, the courage to stand back up when things seemed futile, *this* is what I want to give to you. I *want* you to give your life and health another try. I *want* you to succeed, and I don't want you to fall into the trap of all those other unscientific and fake quickie diet programs that have absolutely no research studies or proof to back them up.

And, please listen, honestly, I think one of the most valuable psychological lessons we can learn along the way in this life is that we all have deficits. We have strengths too, but it is amazing to realize that in overcoming our deficits that is usually what makes us rise up, and this is what keeps our hearts pure enough to then in return *want* to help others. To this day, I honor compassion and humility as the greatest gifts of our Creator.

You may not have that support system, that love that you needed back then, but we are a team now, a family now. I want you to come read, come play, come learn, come heal, and come achieve. You are safe here. I am here to stand tall and tell you in no uncertain terms, if you have ever been told you are not good enough, think to yourself, thank God, and don't listen. There is not only a special path for you but one that brings you the health and appreciation for a physically healthy body and gives you your energetic life back in return.

Cheers to the beauty of nature for knowing what we need more than we know ourselves and to the magic that happens in the cycle of life we are currently in. When we discover that the mind, body, and spirit are one and that with the proper information and recent discoveries I have been blessed to "stumble upon" with great commitment and effort, we can all go out and live balanced, nutritionally supportive versus depletive lifestyles, which will lead us into the longevity of optimal health and peak performance.

All I can truly say is thank you. Thank you from the depths of my soul for taking this journey with me. I hope to see you along the future paths as they evolve and know that I am here to serve in whatever capacity can help the most people.

And, finally in closing, as the archer would tell his apprentice (student), you have been well trained (grasshopper). Now it is time to go and *hit your mark*! And with the universal ripple effect of the heart that works in gratitude, the mind in clarity, and the spirit in truth, we *can* change the world.

What an honor it is that I am finally able to share the gifts that have been given to me, the ones that for a long time, even I could not see. What a wild ride these five and a half decades have taken me on, but now that I know as an "archer" my job is to train *you* to keep your eyes on the PRISE. I do believe the evolution of nutrition and applied physiology has just begun! Now, with the skills to achieve, we need only to believe.

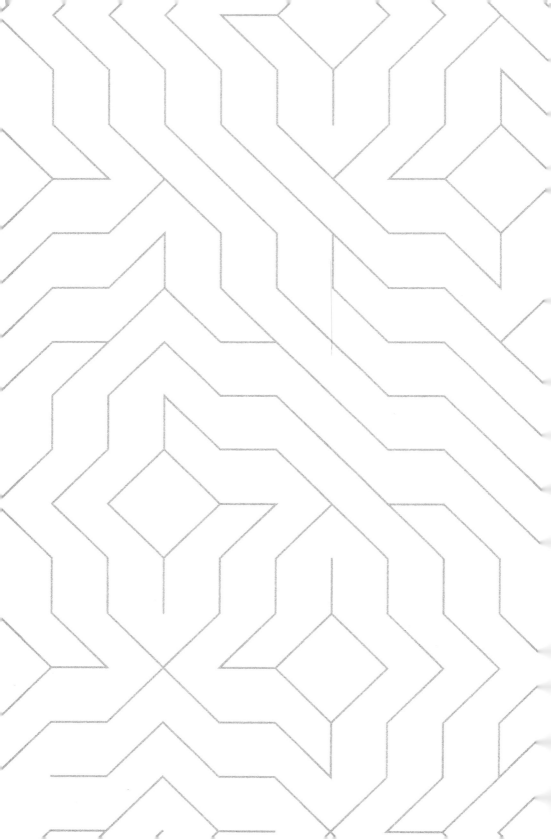

My Eternal Devotion and Gratitude
Thank you for the memories…

To Grandpa John Petrillo, Grandma Deedie Arciero, Donald Vincent Arciero, Jane Barbara (Petrillo) Arciero

My mother, Jane Barbara (Petrillo) Arciero (a vibrant and active nurturer—"The eighty-four-year-old hiking grandma"), who, along with my father, Donald Vincent Arciero ("Big D," your spirit lives on forever for living every day with humility and grace), you were at the forefront of living a life of optimal health and peak performance. You inspired my earliest entry into the field of nutrition, fitness, and health and created my *essence* of being.

My grandfather, John Petrillo, and grandmother, Edith (Deedie) Dean Arciero. You gave me constant love and always believed in me when I didn't always believe in myself. Your legacies live on in me and my family every day.

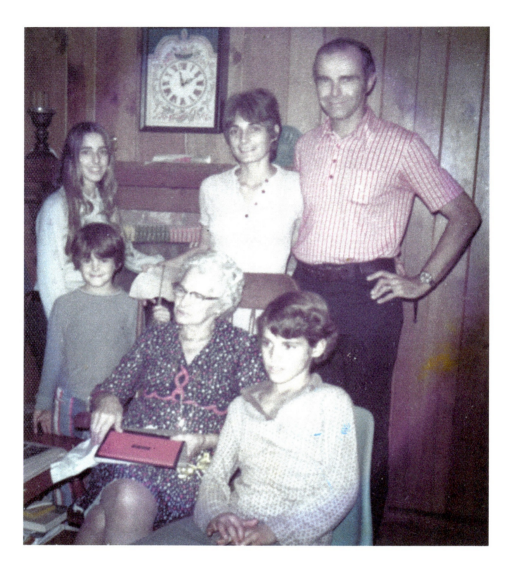

Paternal "Grandma Deedie" Arciero sitting with me (front center). My mom, Jane Barbara (Petrillo) Arciero, "The eighty-four-year-old hiking grandma," and dad, Donald Vincent Arciero ("Big D"), are standing behind us, along with my oldest sister Donna and youngest brother Matt.

Mon. am.
Jan 20, 75

Dear Paul,

I have about six letters to write today and yours is the first. You certainly are very special with me, so thought I'd do yours before I got too tired.

Being in the hospital over the holidays I didn't send Christmas greetings to many of my

friends and relative
so have to let them
know the reason.

It's good to be back in
my little apartment.
and I have very nice
neighbors.

Sorry the pjs got sort
of mixed up but you see
I had purchased them
before I went to the Doc
and when I had to go
right to the hospital
your cousin Denise
who is a Student nurse
up at N. R. volontered
to wrap them. I also
had Christmas card
but forgot to tell her
so it's here and I'll
get it up to you all
as soon as I can.

Give my love to your

Mom, Dad, sisters and brothers.. Thank you, again for your nice letter. Lots of love. Grandma Deedie

Grandma Deedie shares how "special" I am to her. A defining moment in my life: A time when I was not "feeling it."

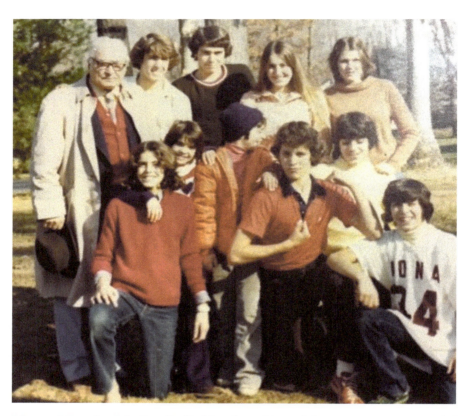

Maternal Grandpa John Petrillo (Left) with me (Center) flexing my arms, surrounded by wonderful siblings and cousins.

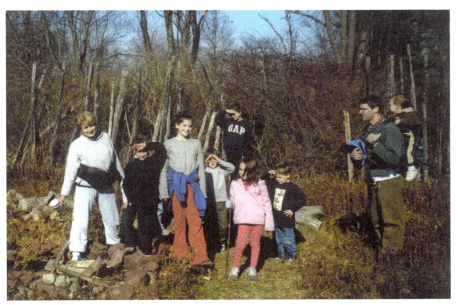

My mom, Jane Barbara (Petrillo) Arciero, (Left) now known by audiences as "The eighty-four-year-old hiking grandma." She is with a small number of her twenty-five total grandkids and four great-grandkids out gardening in the woods. My two older sons are in this picture along with some cousins.

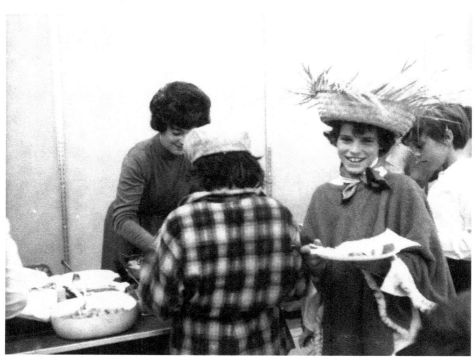

Me on "Food Day" in fifth grade representing the country of Argentina. You can see the pure joy in my smile as a result of my newfound appreciation of healthy eating that was developed from gardening with my mom.

Bibliography

2017. http://www.askdrsears.com/topics/feeding-eating/ family-nutrition/ standard-american-diet-sad

2017. https://bionutrient.org/sites/all/files/docs/2011_ Nutrient_Guide.pdf

2017. http://www.wellnessresources.com/weight/articles/ why-toxins-and-waste-products-impede-weight-loss-theleptin-diet-weight "II. Dynamics of Fat Metabolism." *How Fat Works*. doi:10.4159/9780674045323-004.

"AAAS—The World's Largest General Scientific Society |." AAAS—The World's Largest General Scientific Society |. March 15, 1970. Accessed February 17, 2018. https://www.aaas.org/https://www.aaas.org/sites/default/files/Agencies.

"A better way to exercise." Skidmore College. Accessed November 24, 2017. http://www.skidmore.edu/news/2014/092314-a-better-way-to-exercise.php.

"ACSM | History." American College of Sports Medicine. Accessed February 23, 2018. http://www.acsm.org/about-acsm/who-we-are/history.

"ACSM | OMHA Reference Search—Chronological Search by Author." American College of Sports Medicine. Accessed February 23, 2018. http://www.acsm.org/public-information/health-physical-activity-reference-database/omha-reference-search---chronological-search-by-author.

"A Sleepless Night Can Wreck Your DNA." Daily Mail (London), July 23, 2015.

Allport, Susan. *The Queen of Fats: Why Omega-3s Were Removed from the Western Diet and What We Can Do to Replace Them*. Berkeley, CA: University of California Press, 2006.

"Abraham-Hicks Publications." Home of Abraham-Hicks Law of Attraction—It All Started Here! Accessed January 14, 2018. http://www.abraham-hicks.com/lawofattractionsource/index.php?i=4.

"Abraham-Hicks Sessions." Abraham-Hicks Sessions. Accessed February 1, 2018. https://abrahamhickssessions.wordpress.com//2014/07/11/metabolism-is-vibrational-response-2/.

Anderson, E. N. *Everyone Eats: Understanding Food and Culture*. 2nd ed. New York: New York University Press, 2014. Anderson-Hanley, Cay, and Paul Arciero. "Seniors Cybercycling for Enhanced Cognitive Performance." *PsycEXTRA Dataset*. doi:10.1037/e530522011-009.

Anderson-Hanley C., Paul J. Arciero, Nicole Barcelos, Joseph Nimon, Tracey Rocha, Marisa Thurin and Molly Maloney. "Executive function and self-regulated exergaming adherence among older adults." *Frontiers in Human Neuroscience*. Dec. 2014; Volume8, Article 989.

Anderson-Hanley, C., P. J. Arciero, A. M. Brickman, J. P. Nimon, N. Okuma, S. C. Westen, M. E. Merz, B. D. Pence, J. A. Woods, A. F. Kramer, and E. A. Zimmerman. "Exergaming and older adult cognition: a cluster randomized clinical trial." *American Journal of Preventive Medicine*. February 2012. Accessed March 20, 2018. https://www.ncbi.nlm.nih.gov/pubmed/22261206.

Anshel, Mark H. *Applied Exercise Psychology: A Practitioner's Guide to Improving Client Health and Fitness*. New York: Springer Publishing Company, 2006.

Aragon, Alan A. Brad J. Schoenfeld, Robert Wildman, Susan Kleiner, Trisha VanDusseldorp, Lem Taylor, Conrad P. Earnest, Paul J. Arciero, Colin Wilborn, Douglas S. Kalman, Jeffrey R. Stout, Darryn S. Willoughby, Bill Campbell, Shawn M. Arent, Laurent Bannock, Abbie E. Smith-Ryan and Jose Antonio. "International society of sports nutrition position stand: Diets and Body Composition." *J Int Soc Sports Nutr.* 201714:16. DOI: 10.1186/s12970-017-0174-y.

"Arciero P - PubMed - NCBI." National Center for Biotechnology Information. Accessed March 16, 2018. https://www.ncbi.nlm.nih.gov/pubmed/?term=arciero%2Bp.

Arciero, Paul. "GenioFit on the App Store." App Store. July 08, 2016. Accessed January 8, 2018. https://itunes.apple.com/us/app/geniofit/id1087668497?mt=8. The 2018 App is now PRISE Fitness App (www.prisewell.com).

Arciero, PJ, et al. "Effects of caffeine ingestion on NE kinetics, fat oxidation, and energy expenditure in younger and older men." *Am. J. Physiol.* 268 (*Endocrinol. Metab.* 31): E1192-E1198 1995.

Arciero PJ, Baur D, Connelly S, Ormsbee MJ. "Timed-daily ingestion of whey protein and exercise training reduces visceral adipose tissue mass and improves insulin resistance: the PRISE study." *J Appl Physiol* (1985). 2014 Jul 1;117(1):1-10

Arciero, PJ. Christopher L. Bougopoulos, Bradley C. Nindl, and Neal L. Benowitz. "Influence of Age on the Thermic Response to Caffeine in Women." *Metabolism*, Vol 49, No 1 (January), 2000: pp 101-107.

Arciero PJ, Edmonds RC, Bunsawat K, Gentile CL, Ketcham C, Darin C, Renna M, Zheng Q, Zhang JZ, Ormsbee MJ. "Protein-Pacing from Food or Supplementation Improves Physical Performance in Overweight Men and Women: The PRISE 2 Study." *Nutrients.* 2016 May 11;8(5)

Arciero, Paul J., and Michael J. Ormsbee. "Relationship of blood pressure, behavioral mood state, and physical activity following caffeine ingestion in younger and older women." *Applied Physiology, Nutrition, and Metabolism* 34, no. 4 (2009): 754-62. doi:10.1139/h09-068.

Arciero, PJ, et al. "Relationship of blood pressure, heart rate and behavioral mood state to norepinephrine kinetics in younger and older men following caffeine ingestion." *European Journal of Clinical Nutrition* 52, no. 11 (1998): 805-12. doi:10.1038/sj.ejcn.1600651.

Arciero PJ, Gentile CL, Martin-Pressman R, Ormsbee MJ, Everett M, Zwicky L, Steele CA. "Increased dietary protein and combined high intensity aerobic and resistance exercise improves body fat distribution and cardiovascular risk factors." *Int J Sport Nutr Exerc Metab.* 2006 Aug;16(4):373-92.

Arciero PJ, Gentile CL, Pressman R, Everett M, Ormsbee MJ, Martin J, Santamore J, Gorman L, Fehling PC, Vukovich MD, Nindl BC. "Moderate protein intake improves total and regional body composition and insulin sensitivity in overweight adults." *Metabolism.* 2008 Jun;57(6):757-65.

Arciero, PJ, et al. "Resting metabolic rate is lower in women than in men." *Journal of Applied Physiology* 75, no. 6 (1993): 2514-520. doi:10.1152/jappl.1993.75.6.2514.

Arciero PJ, Hannibal NS, Nindl BC, Gentile CL, Hamed J, Vukovich MD. "Comparison of creatine ingestion and resistance training on energy expenditure and limb blood flow." *Metabolism: Clinical and Experimental*, vol 50: pp 1429-1434, 2001.

Arciero PJ, Ives SJ, Norton C, Escudero D, Minicucci O, O'Brien G, Paul M, Ormsbee MJ, Miller V, Sheridan C, He F. "Protein-Pacing and Multi-Component Exercise Training Improves Physical Performance Outcomes in Exercise-Trained Women: The PRISE 3 Study." *Nutrients*. 2016 Jun 1;8(6)

Arciero PJ, Miller VJ, Ward E. "Performance Enhancing Diets and the PRISE Protocol to Optimize Athletic Performance." *J Nutr Metab*. 2015;2015:715859

Arciero PJ, Ormsbee MJ, Gentile CL, Nindl BC, Brestoff JR, Ruby M. "Increased protein intake and meal frequency reduces abdominal fat during energy balance and energy deficit." *Obesity* (Silver Spring). 2013 Jul;21(7):1357-66

Arciero PJ, Smith DL, Calles-Escandon J. "Effects of inactivity on glucose tolerance, energy expenditure and blood flow in highly trained endurance athletes." *J Appl Physiol*, 1998; 84:1217-1224.

Arciero PJ, Vukovich MD, Holloszy JO, Racette S, Kohrt WM. "Comparison of a short-term diet and exercise training on insulin action in individuals with abnormal glucose tolerance." *J Appl Physiol*. 86(6): 1930-1935, 1999.

Arciero, Paul, Rohan Edmonds, Feng He, Emery Ward, Eric Gumpricht, Alex Mohr, Michael Ormsbee, and Arne Astrup. "Protein-Pacing Caloric-Restriction Enhances Body Composition Similarly in Obese Men and Women during Weight Loss and Sustains Efficacy during Long-Term Weight Maintenance." *Nutrients* 8, no. 8 (2016): 476. doi:10.3390/nu8080476.

Areta, J.L.; Burke, L.M.; Camera, D.M. ;West, D.W.; Crawshay, S.; Moore, D.R.; Stellingwerff, T.; Phillips, S.M.; Hawley, J.A.; Coffey, V.G. "Reduced resting skeletal muscle protein synthesis is rescued by resistance exercise and protein ingestion following short-term energy deficit." *Am. J. Physiol. Endocrinol. Metab*. 2014, 306, 989–997.

Astrup, A.; Raben, A.; Geiker, N. "The role of higher protein diets in weight control and obesity-related comorbidities." *Int. J. Obes*. 2014, 39, 721–726.

Bajarin, Tim. "Fitbit: Here's Why Fitness Trackers Are Here to Stay." *Time*. June 24, 2015. Accessed March 3, 2018. http://time.com/3934258/ fitness-trackers-fitbit/?xid=emailshare.

Barcelos, Nicole, Nikita Shah, Katherine Cohen, Michael J. Hogan, Eamon Mulkerrin, Paul J. Arciero, Brian D. Cohen, Arthur F. Kramer and Cay Anderson-Hanley. "Aerobic and Cognitive Exercise (ACE) Pilot Study for Older Adults: Executive Function Improves with Cognitive Challenge While Exergaming." *JINS*, 21: 10; 768-779, 2015.

Barrett, Julia R. "The Science of Soy: What Do We Really Know?" *Environmental Health Perspectives* 114, no. 6 (2006): A352+.

Batacan, Romeo B., Mitch J. Duncan, Vincent J. Dalbo, Patrick S. Tucker, and Andrew S. Fenning. "Effects of high-intensity interval training on cardiometabolic health: a systematic review and meta-analysis of intervention studies." *British Journal of Sports Medicine* 51, no. 6 (2016): 494-503. doi:10.1136/bjsports-2015-095841.

Baum, J. I., M. Gray, and A. Binns. "Breakfasts Higher in Protein Increase Postprandial Energy Expenditure, Increase Fat Oxidation, and Reduce Hunger in Overweight Children from 8 to 12 Years of Age." *The Journal of Nutrition*. October 2015. Accessed January 22, 2018. https://www.ncbi.nlm.nih.gov/pubmed/26269241.

Berardi, Ph.D. John. "Breakfast: Not Really the Most Important Meal of the Day." *The Huffington Post*. December 15, 2013. Accessed March 18, 2018. https://www. huffingtonpost.com/john-berardi-phd/breakfast-health_b_4436439.html.

Berger, Vance W., and A. J. Sankoh. "Prognostic Variables in Clinical Trials." *Methods and Applications of Statistics in Clinical Trials*, 2014, 789-98. doi:10.1002/9781118596005.ch67.

Bergman, Bryan C., Leigh Perreault, Allison Strauss, Samantha Bacon, Anna Kerege, Kathleen Harrison, Joseph T. Brozinick, Devon M. Hunerdosse, Mary C. Playdon, William Holmes, Hai Hoang Bui, Phil Sanders, Parker Siddall, Tao Wei, Melissa K. Thomas, Ming Shang Kuo, and Robert H. Eckel. "Intramuscular triglyceride synthesis: importance in muscle lipid partitioning in humans." *American Journal of Physiology-Endocrinology and Metabolism* 314, no. 2 (2018). doi:10.1152/ajpendo.00142.2017.

"Best Way to Slow Aging? High-Intensity Interval Training Exercise—but Not Just Any Kind." *The Buffalo News* (Buffalo, NY), April 15, 2017.

"Biochemistry & Molecular Biology." *Michigan Academician* 37, no. 4 (2008): 10+.

Boecker, H., T. Sprenger, M. E. Spilker, G. Henriksen, M. Koppenhoefer, K. J. Wagner, M. Valet, A. Berthele, and T. R. Tolle. "The runners high: opioidergic mechanisms in the human brain." *Cerebral Cortex* (New York, NY:1991). November 2008. Accessed March 20, 2018. https://www.ncbi.nlm.nih.gov/pubmed/18296435.

Bugaut, M. "Occurrence, Absorption and Metabolism of Short Chain Fatty Acids in the Digestive Tract of Mammals." *Comparative Biochemistry and Physiology. B, Comparative Biochemistry*. Accessed March 5, 2018. https://www.ncbi.nlm.nih.gov/pubmed/3297476.

Burke, Louise, and Greg Cox. *The Complete Guide to Food for Sports Performance: A Guide to Peak Nutrition for Your Sport*. 3rd ed. Crow's Nest, N.S.W.: Allen & Unwin, 2010.

"CDC Newsroom." Centers for Disease Control and Prevention. July 18, 2017. Accessed February 23, 2018. https://www.cdc.gov/media/releases/2017/p0718-diabetes-report.html.

"Carbohydrates and Resistant Starch May Help Weight Loss." *Time*. Accessed November 22, 2017. http://time.com/4318201/carbohydrates-weight-loss-resistant-starch/.

Case, Meredith A. "Accuracy of Devices to Track Physical Activity Data." *JAMA*. February 10, 2015. Accessed March 3, 2018. https://jamanetwork.com/journals/jama/fullarticle/2108876#tab1.

Centers for Disease Control and Prevention. June 02, 2009. Accessed February 18, 2018. https://www.cdc.gov/nchs/data/hus/hus16.pdf#056.

Chaput, J-P Després, C. Bouchard, and A. Tremblay. "Longer sleep duration associates with lower adiposity gain in adult short sleepers." *Nature News*. June 07, 2011. Accessed March 1, 2018. http://www.nature.com/articles/ijo2011110.

Chaput, Jean-Philippe, Jessica McNeilJean-Pierre Després, Claude Bouchard, and Angelo Tremblay. "Seven to Eight Hours of Sleep a Night Is Associated with a Lower Prevalence of the Metabolic Syndrome and Reduced Overall Cardiometabolic Risk in Adults." PLOS ONE. Accessed March 11, 2018. http://journals.plos.org/plosone/article?id=10.1371%2Fjournal.pone.0072832.

Cheeke, P. R., and E. S. Dierenfeld. "Fat and fatty acid metabolism." Comparative animal nutrition and metabolism: 133-44. doi:10.1079/9781845936310.0133.

Cheikh Rouhou, M.; Karelis, A.D.; St-Pierre, D.H.; Lamontagne, L. "Adverse effects of weight loss: Are persistent organic pollutants a potential culprit?" *Diabetes Metab*. 2016, 42, 215–223.

Chivian, Eric, Aaron Bernstein, and Kofi Annan, eds. *Sustaining Life: How Human Health Depends on Biodiversity*. New York: Oxford University Press, 2008.

"Clean Your Body's Drains: 10 Ways to Detoxify Your Lymphatic System." 2017. Healthy and Natural World. http://www.healthyandnaturalworld.com/ natural-ways-to-cleanse-your-lymphatic-system/

Clifton, P.M.; Bastiaans, K.; Keogh, J.B. "High protein diets decrease total and abdominal fat and improve CVD risk profile in overweight and obese men and women with elevated triacylglycerol." *Nutr. Metab. Cardiovasc. Dis.* 2009, 19, 548–554.

Connor, Erinn. "Be Aware of the Sleep-Weight Connections." *The Record* (Bergen County, NJ), March 7, 2013.

Cotterill, Stewart. *Team Psychology in Sports: Theory and Practice.* New York: Routledge, 2012.

Cui, Yufei, Kaijun Niu, Cong Huang, Haruki Momma, Lei Guan, Hui Guo, Masahiko Chujo, Atsushi Otomo, and Ryoichi Nagatomi. "Relationship between daily isoflavone intake and sleep in Japanese adults: a cross-sectional study." *Nutrition Journal.* December 29, 2015. Accessed March 3, 2018. https://nutritionj.biomedcentral.com/articles/10.1186/ s12937-015-0117-x.

"Dairy Processing Handbook." Dairy Processing Handbook. Accessed February 11, 2018. http://dairyprocessinghandbook.com/chapter/whey-processing.

Diamond, Dan. "Just 8% of People Achieve Their New Year's Resolutions. Here's How They Do It." Forbes. January 02, 2013. Accessed January 14, 2018. https://www.forbes.com/sites/dandiamond/2013/01/01/ just-8-of-people-achieve-their-new-years-resolutions-heres-how-they-did-it/2/.

"Dimethyl Sulfoxide (DMSO) and Methylsulfonylmethane (MSM) for Osteoarthritis." National Center for Complementary and Integrative Health. September 24, 2017. Accessed February 23, 2018. https://nccih.nih.gov/health/supplements/dmso-msm.

Dansinger, M.L.; Gleason, J.A.; Griffith, J.L.; Selker, H.P.; Schaefer, E.J. "Comparison of the Atkins, Ornish, Weight Watchers, and Zone diets for weight loss and heart disease risk reduction: A randomized trial." *J. Am. Med. Assoc.* 2005, 293, 43–53.

"Definition." American Society of Exercise Physiologists. Accessed December 18, 2017. https://www.asep.org/about-asep/definition/.

"Digesting 'Fat Chance' and Understanding Obesity." *Daily Herald* (Arlington Heights, IL), January 30, 2013.

"Digital Object Identifier System." Digital Object Identifier System. Accessed December 19, 2017. https://doi.org/10.1080/00336297.2007.10483534.

"Dr. Arciero: Losing Weight & Keeping it Off - Isagenix Podcast." The Official Isagenix Podcast Site. August 11, 2017. Accessed November 24, 2017. http://isagenixpodcast. com/dr-arciero-losing-weight-keeping-off/.

"Dr. Paul Arciero, Skidmore College." WAMC. Accessed November 28, 2017. http://wamc. org/post/dr-paul-arciero-skidmore-college.

DrPaulsProtocol. "Dr. Paul Arciero." YouTube. Accessed November 25, 2017. http://www. youtube.com/user/DrPaulsProtocol.

Dirinck, E.L.; Dirtu, A.C.; Govindan, M.; Covaci, A.; Jorens, P.G.; van Gaal, L.F. "Endocrine-disrupting polychlorinated biphenyls in metabolically healthy and unhealthy obese subjects before and after weight loss: Difference at the start but not at the finish." *Am. J. Clin. Nutr.* 2016, 103, 989–998.

Dirinck, E.; Dirtu, A.C.; Jorens, P.G.; Malarvannan, G.; Covaci, A.; Van Gaal, L.F. "Pivotal role for the visceral fat compartment in the release of persistent organic pollutants during weight loss." *J. Clin. Endocrinol. Metab.* 2015, 100, 4463–4471.

DrugWatch. July 29, 2015. Accessed January 8, 2018. https://www.drugwatch. com/2015/07/29/drug-abuse-in-america/.

"Eating More Can Help You to Lose Weight. Understand Your Body and Change Your Life." *Daily Mail* (London), April 14, 1997.

"Eight Eating Habits You Need to Break." *The Buffalo News* (Buffalo, NY), August 22, 2015.

Elder, Charles R., Christina M. Gullion, Kristine L. Funk, Lynn L. DeBar, Nangel M. Lindberg, and Victor J. Stevens. *International Journal of Obesity* (2005). January 2012. Accessed March 20, 2018. https://www.ncbi.nlm.nih.gov/pmc/articles/PMC3136584/.

Elkins, Chris. "Hooked on Pharmaceuticals: Prescription Drug Abuse in America."

Evans, Malkanthi, John Rumberger, Isao Azumano, Joseph Napolitano, Danielle Citrolo, and Toshikazu Kamiya. "Pantethine, a derivative of vitamin B5, favorably alters total, LDL and non-HDL cholesterol in low to moderate cardiovascular risk subjects eligible for statin therapy: a triple-blinded placebo and diet-controlled investigation." *Vascular Health and Risk Management*, 2014, 89. doi:10.2147/vhrm.s57116.

"EXERCISE PHYSIOLOGY." Ece Soccer. Accessed December 15, 2017. http://ece-soccer.com/dt_activities/physiology/.

"Exergaming and Older Adult Cognition: A Cluster Randomized Clinical Trial." *American Journal of Preventive Medicine*. January 16, 2012. Accessed March 20, 2018. https://www.sciencedirect.com/science/article/pii/S0749379711008622.

Farahbakhsh-Farsi, Payam, Abolghassem Djazayery, Mohammad Reza Eshraghian, Fariba Koohdani, Mahnaz Zarei, Mohammad Hassan Javanbakht, Hoda Derakhshanian, and Mahmoud Djalali. "Effect of Omega-3 Supplementation on Lipocalin 2 and Retinol-Binding Protein 4 in Type 2 Diabetic Patients." *Iranian Journal of Public Health* 45, no. 1 (2016): 63+.

"Fat and Calories." Cleveland Clinic. Accessed January 9, 2018. https://my.clevelandclinic.org/health/articles/4182-fat-and-calories.

"Fat May Spur Heart Cells on to Suicide." *Science News*, May 12, 2001.

Feudtner, Chris. *Bittersweet: Diabetes, Insulin, and the Transformation of Illness*. Edited by Allan M. Brandt and Larry R. Churchill. Chapel Hill, NC: University of North Carolina Press, 2003.

"Fiber and Saturated Fat Are Associated with Sleep Arousals and Slow Wave." National Center for Biotechnology Information. Accessed March 3, 2018. https://www.ncbi.nlm.nih.gov/pubmed.

Fossel, Michael B. *Cells, Aging, and Human Disease*. New York: Oxford University Press, 2004.

Franz, M.J.; Van Wormer, J.J.; Crain, A.L.; Boucher, J.L.; Histon, T.; Caplan, W.; Bowman, J.D.; Pronk, N.P. "Weight-loss outcomes: A systematic review and meta-analysis of weight-loss clinical trials with a minimum 1-year follow-up." *J. Am. Diet. Assoc.* 2007, 107, 1755–1767.

Gaidos, Susan. "Fat as a Fixer: Adipose Tissue Is a Natural Storehouse of Healing Cells." *Science News*, March 19, 2016, 22+.

Gardner, C.D.; Kiazand, A.; Alhassan, S.; Kim, S.; Stafford, R.S.; Balise, R.R.; Kraemer, H.C.; King, A.C. "Comparison of the Atkins, Zone, Ornish, and LEARN diets for change in weight and related risk factors among overweight premenopausal women: The A TO Z Weight Loss Study: A randomized trial." *J. Am. Med. Assoc.* 2007, 297, 969–977.

Gardner, C. D., J. F. Trepanowski, L. C. Del, M. E. Hauser, J. Rigdon, J. P. Ioannidis, M. Desai, and A. C. King. "Effect of Low-Fat vs Low-Carbohydrate Diet on 12-Month Weight Loss in Overweight Adults and the Association with Genotype Pattern or Insulin Secretion: The DIETFITS Randomized Clinical Trial." *JAMA*. February 20, 2018. Accessed March 26, 2018. https://www.ncbi.nlm.nih.gov/pubmed/29466592.

"GenioFit—The guide to get you there." GenioFit. Accessed November 24, 2017. http://www.geniofit.com/. The 2018 App is now PRISE Fitness App (www.prisewell.com).

Genné-Bacon, Elizabeth A. *The Yale Journal of Biology and Medicine*. June 2014. Accessed January 18, 2018. https://www.ncbi.nlm.nih.gov/pmc/articles/PMC4031802/.

Gentile, Christopher L., Emery Ward, Jens Juul Holst, Arne Astrup, Michael J. Ormsbee, Scott Connelly, and Paul J. Arciero. "Resistant starch and protein intake enhances fat oxidation and feelings of fullness in lean and overweight/obese women." *Nutrition Journal*. October 29, 2015. Accessed January 20, 2018. https://nutritionj.biomedcentral.com/articles/10.1186/s12937-015-0104-2.

Gibbons, Ann, and Matthieu Paley. "The Evolution of Diet." *National Geographic*. Accessed January 18, 2018. https://www.nationalgeographic.com/foodfeatures/evolution-of-diet/.

Gluckman, Peter, and Mark Hanson. *Mismatch: Why Our World No Longer Fits Our Bodies*. New York: Oxford University Press, 2006.

Goho, Alexandra. "Our Microbes, Ourselves: How Bacterial Communities in the Body Influence Human Health." *Science News*, May 19, 2007, 314+.

"GoodTherapy.org." Erik Erikson Biography. Accessed January 8, 2018. https://www.goodtherapy.org/famous-psychologists/erik-erikson.html.

Google. Accessed March 17, 2018. https://scholar.google.com/scholar?start=0&q=arciero pj&hl=en&as_sdt=0,3.

Grey, Jennie. "Students in Saratoga Springs High school's new nutrition class tour Skidmore College labs." *The Saratogian*. October 22, 2012. Accessed March 10, 2018. http://www.saratogian.com/article/ST/20121022/NEWS/310229936.

"Guide to Healthy Drinks." www.be-fit.me. Accessed March 10, 2018. http://www.be-fit.me/guide-to-healthy-drinks-411/.

Harris, Herbert W., Pranay Jaiswal, Valerie Holmes, Richard H. Weisler, and Ashwin A. Patkar. "Vitamin D Deficiency and Psychiatric Illness: Supplementation Might Help Patients with Depression, Seasonal Mood Disturbances." *Current Psychiatry* 12, no. 4 (2013): 18+.

He, Feng, Li Zuo, Emery Ward, and Paul Arciero. "Serum Polychlorinated Biphenyls Increase and Oxidative Stress Decreases with a Protein-Pacing Caloric Restriction Diet in Obese Men and Women." *International Journal of Environmental Research and Public Health* 14, no. 12 (2017): 59. doi:10.3390/ijerph14010059.

Health A-Z. Accessed January 9, 2018. http://www.betterlifeunlimited.com/healthnews/health_az/issues/macronutrients_carbohydrates_proteins_and_fats.aspx.

Hefferon, Kathleen. *Let Thy Food Be Thy Medicine: Plants and Modern Medicine*. New York: Oxford University Press, 2012.

Heymsfield, S.B.; Harp, J.B.; Reitman, M.L.; Beetsch, J.W.; Schoeller, D.A.; Erondu, N.; Pietrobelli, A. "Why do obese patients not lose more weight when treated with low-calorie diets? A mechanistic perspective." *Am. J. Clin. Nutr.* 2007, 85, 346–354.

"History of Psychology (387 BC to Present)." AllPsych. Accessed February 22, 2018. https://allpsych.com/timeline/.

Hopper, Christopher A., Bruce Fisher, and Kathy D. Munoz. *Physical Activity and Nutrition for Health*. Champaign, IL: Human Kinetics, 2008.

"How to exercise less and get better results." All 4 Women. June 03, 2014. Accessed March 10, 2018. https://www.all4women.co.za/211583/health/how-to-exercise-less-and-get-better-results.

"How to get into the best shape of your life, according to science." Fox News. Accessed March 10, 2018. http://www.foxnews.com/lifestyle/2017/04/06/how-to-get-into-best-shape-your-life-according-to-science.html.

Howell, S., and R. Kones. "Calories In, Calories Out" and Macronutrient Intake: The Hope, Hype, and Science of Calories." *American Journal of Physiology, Endocrinology and Metabolism*. November 01, 2017. Accessed March 26, 2018. https://www.ncbi.nlm.nih.gov/pubmed/28765272.

Hunter, Beatrice Trum. "The Form Counts: Proteins, Fats and Carbohydrates." *Consumers' Research Magazine*, August 2001.

Imbeault, P.; Tremblay, A.; Simoneau, J.A.; Joanisse, D.R. "Weight loss-induced rise in plasma pollutant is associated with reduced skeletal muscle oxidative capacity." *Am. J. Physiol. Endocrinol. Metab.* 2002, 282, E574–E579.

"Inflammation and Its Diseases." *Nutrition Health Review*, January 1, 2013, 2+.

"Is breakfast really the most important meal? Why a new study says maybe not." TODAY.com. Accessed March 18, 2018. https://www.today.com/health/new-study-says-breakfast-may-not-be-most-important-meal-t37991.

"Is Soy Bad for You?—Dr. Axe." 2017. Dr. Axe. https:// draxe.com/is-soy-bad-for-you/

Ives SJ, Bloom S, Matias A, Morrow N, Martins N, Roh Y, Ebenstein D, O'Brien G, Escudero D, Brito K, Glickman L, Connelly S, Arciero PJ (Senior Corresponding Author). "Effects of a combined protein and antioxidant supplement on recovery of muscle function and soreness following eccentric exercise." *J Int Soc Sports Nutr*. 2017 Jul 3;14:21.

Ives SJ, Norton C, Miller V, Minicucci O, Robinson J, O'Brien G, Escudero D, Paul M, Sheridan C, Curran K, Rose K, Robinson N, He F, Arciero PJ. "Multi-modal exercise training and protein-pacing enhances physical performance adaptations independent of growth hormone and BDNF but may be dependent on IGF-1 in exercise-trained men." Growth Horm IGF Res. 2017 Feb;32:60-70.

R. Jäger, et al. . "International Society of Sports Nutrition Position Stand: Protein and Exercise." *J Int Soc Sports Nutr*. 2017 14:20 DOI: 10.1186/s12970-017-0177-8.

Jahnke, Art. "Who Picks Up the Tab for Science?" History and Future of Funding for Scientific   Research | Research. Accessed January 8, 2018. http://www.bu.edu/research/articles/funding-for-scientific-research/.

Jeffers, Glenn. "Training for a Marathon. (Body Talk: Black Health and Fitness)." *Ebony*, March 2003, 86+.

Johansen, Bruce E. *The Dirty Dozen: Toxic Chemicals and the Earth's Future*. Westport, CT: Praeger, 2003.

Kadey, Matthew. "Attack of the Diet Saboteurs." *Vegetarian Times*, January/February 2015, 70+.

Kelli, Heval Mohamed, Frank Corrigan, Robert Heinl, Devinder Dhindsa, Muhammad Hammadah, Ayman Samman-Tahhan, Pratik Sandesara, Talal Alghamdi, Ibhar Al Mheid, Yi-An Ko, Thomas Ziegler, Laurence Sperling, Kenneth Brigham, Dean Jones, Viola Vaccarino, Greg Martin, and Arshed Quyyumi. "Changes in Body Fat Distribution Is Associated with Oxidative Stress." *Journal of the American College of Cardiology* 69, no. 11 (2017): 1795. doi:10.1016/s0735-1097(17)35184-7.

Kerksick, Chad; Shawn Arent; Brad J Schoenfeld; Jeffrey R Stout; Bill Campbell; Colin Wilborn; Lem Taylor; Doug Kalman; Abbie E Smith-Ryan; Richard B Kreider; Darryn Willoughby; Paul J. Arciero; Trisha VanDusseldorp; Mike Ormsbee; Robert Wildman; Mike Greenwood; Tim Ziegenfuss; Alan A Aragon; Jose Antonio. "International Society of Sports Nutrition Position Stand: Nutrient Timing." *J Int Soc Sports Nutr.* 14:33 https://doi.org/10.1186/s12970-017-0189-4.

Kinsey, A. W., Eddy, W., Madzima, T., Panton, L., Arciero, P.J., Kim, J-S, & Ormsbee, M. J. "The Influence of Nighttime Protein and Carbohydrate Intake on Appetite and Cardiometabolic Risk in Sedentary Overweight and Obese Women." *Br J Nutr*, 2015. Tyler Graham."Laird Hamilton's Bulletproof Coffee Breakfast Recipe." *Men's Journal.* December 05, 2017. Accessed March 10, 2018. https://www.mensjournal.com/health-fitness/bulletproof-coffee-the-new-power-breakfast-20141117/.

Larsen, T.M.; Dalskov, S.; van Baak, M.; Jebb, S.A.; Papadaki, A.; Pfeiffer, A.F.H.; Martinez, J.A.; Handjieva-Darlenska, T.; Kunesova, M.; Pihlsgard, M.; et al. "Diets with high or low protein content and glycemic index for weight-loss maintenance." *N. Engl. J. Med.* 2010, 363, 2102–2113.

Lawrence, Glen D. *The Fats of Life: Essential Fatty Acids in Health and Disease.* New Brunswick, NJ: Rutgers University Press, 2010.

"Learn about Dioxin." EPA. March 22, 2017. Accessed February 25, 2018. https://www.epa.gov/dioxin/learn-about-dioxin.

Lees, A., I. Maynard, M. Hughes, and T. Reilly, eds. *Science and Racket Sports II.* London: E & FN Spon, 1998.

Lees, A., J.-F. Kahn, and I. W. Maynard. *Science and Racket Sports III.* New York: Routledge, 2004.

Leidy, H. J., H. A. Hoertel, S. M. Douglas, K. A. Higgins, and R. S. Shafer. "A high-protein breakfast prevents body fat gain, through reductions in daily intake and hunger, in 'Breakfast skipping' adolescents." *Obesity* (Silver Spring, Md.). September 2015. Accessed March 18, 2018. https://www.ncbi.nlm.nih.gov/pubmed/26239831.

Levine, James A. "Non-exercise activity thermogenesis (NEAT)." *Best Practice & Research Clinical Endocrinology & Metabolism* 16, no. 4 (2002): 679-702. doi:10.1053/beem.2002.0227.

MacMillan, Amanda. "Why Athletes Should Use Caffeine Patches." Outside Online. April 12, 2017. Accessed March 10, 2018. https://www.outsideonline.com/1786291/are-caffeine-patches-safe-athletes.

Manninen, Anssi H. *Journal of the International Society of Sports Nutrition.* 2004. Accessed March 3, 2018. https://www.ncbi.nlm.nih.gov/pmc/articles/PMC2129159/.

Manton, Catherine. *Fed Up: Women and Food in America.* Westport, CT: Bergin & Garvey, 1999.

Martarelli, Daniele, Mario Cocchioni, Stefania Scuri, and Pierluigi Pompei. Evidence-based Complementary and Alternative Medicine: eCAM. 2011. Accessed March 20, 2018. https://www.ncbi.nlm.nih.gov/pmc/articles/PMC3139518/.

"Medical News Today." *Medical News Today.* Accessed February 11, 2018. https://www.medicalnewstoday.com/articles/263371.php.

"Meditation-Based Program Unveiled for Tennis Players." *International Journal of Humanities and Peace* 19, no. 1 (2003): 103.

Mednick, Sara C., Nicholas A. Christakis, and James H. Fowler. "The Spread of Sleep Loss Influences Drug Use in Adolescent Social Networks." PLOS ONE. Accessed March 1, 2018. http://journals.plos.org/plosone/article?id=10.1371%2Fjournal.pone.0009775.

"Miracle tricks to burning calories." IOL Lifestyle. November 13, 2016. Accessed March 10, 2018. https://www.iol.co.za/lifestyle/health/miracle-tricks-to-burning-calories-623661.

Mosher, Rachel, Kyler Crawford, and Andrea Lukowiak. "A Soy-Based Alternative to Traditional Bacterial Nutrient Media." *The American Biology Teacher* 71, no. 1 (2009): 49+.

Mozaffarian, Dariush. "US Dietary Guidelines and Lifting the Total Dietary Fat Ban." *JAMA.* June 23, 2015. Accessed February 25, 2018. https://jamanetwork.com/journals/jama/article-abstract/2338262?resultClick=3&redirect=true.

"National Center for Biotechnology Information." National Center for Biotechnology Information. Accessed February 11, 2018. https://www.ncbi.nlm.nih.gov/pmc/articles/PMC3905294/.

"National Center for Health Statistics." Centers for Disease Control and Prevention. March 17, 2017. Accessed February 23, 2018. https://www.cdc.gov/nchs/fastats/leading-causes-of-death.htm.

Nestle, Marion. *Food Politics: How the Food Industry Influences Nutrition and Health.* Revised ed. Berkeley, CA: University of California Press, 2013.

"New Isagenix Study Findings on Weight Loss and Toxins." *Isagenix Health.* March 15, 2017. Accessed November 24, 2017. http://www.isagenixhealth.net/new-isagenix-study-findings-weight-loss-toxins/.

OECD. "OECD Statistics." OECD Statistics. Accessed March 7, 2018. https://stats.oecd.org/.

"Opioid Overdose." Centers for Disease Control and Prevention. August 30, 2017. Accessed January 8, 2018. https://www.cdc.gov/drugoverdose/epidemic/index.html.

Ormsbee MJ & Arciero PJ (Senior Corresponding Author). "Detraining Increases Body Fat and Weight and Decreases VO2peak and Metabolic Rate." *J Strength Cond Res*, 26(8): 2087-2095, 2012.

Ormsbee MJ, Kinsey AW, Eddy WR, Madzima TA, Arciero PJ, Panton LB. "The influence of exercise training and nighttime eating in overweight and obese women." *Appl. Physiol. Nutr. Metab.* 40: 1–9 (2015)

"Overweight & Obesity." Centers for Disease Control and Prevention. August 31, 2017. Accessed February 25, 2018. https://www.cdc.gov/obesity/data/prevalence-maps.html.

"Paul J Arciero." Paul J Arciero - The Obesity Society. Accessed November 24, 2017. http://www.obesity.org/content/paul-arciero.

"Paul J Arciero | Publications - ResearchGate." Accessed November 24, 2017. https://www.bing.com/Paul_Arciero publications,5458.1.

"Paul J. Arciero." Paul J. Arciero. Accessed November 24, 2017. https://www.skidmore.edu/exercisescience/faculty/paul-arciero.php.

Palmore, Erdman B., Frank Whittington, and Suzanne Kunkel, eds. *The International Handbook on Aging: Current Research and Developments*. 3rd ed. Santa Barbara, CA: Praeger, 2009.

Park, Sung Kyun, Joel Schwartz, Marc Weisskopf, David Sparrow, Pantel S. Vokonas,

"Pete Seeger—Keep Your Eyes on the Prize." Genius. Accessed February 16, 2018. https://genius.com/Pete-seeger-keep-your-eyes-on-the-prize-lyrics.

Pogue, David. "Fitness Trackers Are Everywhere, but Do They Work?" *Scientific American*. January 01, 2015. Accessed March 2, 2018. https://www.scientificamerican.com/article/fitness-trackers-are-everywhere-but-do-they-work/.

"PsycNET." American Psychological Association. Accessed January 8, 2018. http://psycnet.apa.org/record/1975-26412-001.

Quantum Emergence System | Dr Matt Mannino. Accessed March 3, 2018. http://quantumemergence.com/qe/.

"Recent Perspectives Regarding the Role of Dietary Protein for the Promotion of Muscle Hypertrophy with Resistance Exercise Training." *Nutrients* 10, no. 2 (2018): 180. doi:10.3390/nu10020180.

Rice, Xan. "Rise of the Super-Agers: As the 100-Year Life Becomes More Common, the Exploits of an Extraordinary Set of Athletes Are Forcing Scientists to Reassess the Relationship between Performance and Growing Old." *New Statesman* (1996), April 7, 2017, 46+.

Robert O. Wright, Brent Coull, Huiling Nie, and Howard Hu. "Low-Level Lead Exposure, Metabolic Syndrome, and Heart Rate Variability: The VA Normative Aging Study." *Environmental Health Perspectives* 114, no. 11 (2006): 1718+.

Rognmo, O., T. Moholdt, H. Bakken, T. Hole, P. Molstad, N. E. Myhr, J. Grimsmo, and U. Wisloff. "Cardiovascular Risk of High-Versus Moderate-Intensity Aerobic Exercise in Coronary Heart Disease Patients." *Circulation* 126, no. 12 (2012): 1436-440. doi:10.1161/circulationaha.112.123117.

Roos, V.; Ronn, M.; Salihovic, S.; Lind, L.; van Bavel, B.; Kullberg, J.; Johansson, L.; Ahlstrom, H.; Lind, P.M. "Circulating levels of persistent organic pollutants in relation to visceral and subcutaneous adipose tissue by abdominal MRI." *Obesity* 2013, 21, 413–418.

Ross, Benjamin, and Steven Amter. *The Polluters: The Making of Our Chemically-Altered Environment*. New York: Oxford University Press, 2010.

Rothblum, Esther, and Sondra Solovay, eds. *The Fat Studies Reader*. New York: New York University Press, 2009.

Ruby M, Repka CP, Arciero PJ. "Comparison of Protein-Pacing Alone or With Yoga/Stretching and Resistance Training on Glycemia, Total and Regional Body Composition, and Aerobic Fitness in Overweight Women." *J Phys Act Health*. 2016 Jul;13(7):754-64

Salvi, Kristin. "Paul Arciero, New York." You're the Cure. Accessed March 10, 2018. https://www.yourethecure.org/paul_arciero_new_york.

"Samples.jbpub.com." Jbpub. Accessed January 8, 2018. http://samples.jbpub.com./9781284034851/Chapter_3.pdf.

ScienceDaily. Accessed November 22, 2017. https://www.sciencedaily.com/releases/2017/01/170111184102.htm.

Scutti, Susan. "A Gut Reaction." *Newsweek*, November 29, 2013.

"Selected Issues for Nutrition and the Athlete: A Team...:Medicine & Science in Sports & Exercise." LWW. Accessed February 2, 2018. https://journals.lww.com/acsm-msse/Fulltext/2013/12000/Selected_Issues_for_Nutrition_and_the_Athlete_A.21.aspx.

Shahzad, Mian M. K., Mildred Felder, Kai Ludwig, Hannah R. Van Galder, Matthew L. Anderson, Jong Kim, Mark E. Cook, Arvinder K. Kapur, and Manish S. Patankar. "Trans10,cis12 conjugated linoleic acid inhibits proliferation and migration of ovarian cancer cells by inducing ER stress, autophagy, and modulation of Src." PLOS ONE. January 11, 2018. Accessed February 23, 2018. http://paperity.org/p/85521415/trans10-cis12-conjugated-linoleic-acid-inhibits-proliferation-and-migration-of-ovarian.

Shearrer, GE, MJ. Daniels, CM. Toledo-Corral, MJ. Weigensberg, D. Spruijt-Metz, and JN. Davis. "Associations among sugar sweetened beverage intake, visceral fat, and cortisol awakening response in minority youth." *Physiology & Behavior* 167 (2016): 188-93. doi:10.1016/j.physbeh.2016.09.020.

"Six Yoga Exercises That Could Change Your Life; Your Life Daily EVERYONE Loves A Quick Fix—Whether It Is to Perfect Your Face, Achieve a Body Beautiful or Whittle Down That Weight. So Wouldn't It Be Great to Be Able to Do Just a Few Simple Exercises a Day to Boost the Body, Mind and Soul? KAREN HAMBRIDGE Investigates. New Year New You." *Coventry Evening Telegraph* (England), January 14, 2008.

Skibola, Christine F., Jianqing Zhang, and Jacques E. Riby. "Heavy Metal Contamination of Powdered Protein and Botanical Shake Mixes." *Journal of Environmental Health* 80, no. 4 (2017): 8+.

"Skidmore and local school students mark National Eating Healthy Day." *The Saratogian.* November 07, 2012. Accessed March 10, 2018. http://www.saratogian.com/article/ST/20121107/NEWS/311079911.

"Skidmore professor headed to Washington to talk about health." NEWS10 ABC. May 11, 2015. Accessed March 10, 2018. http://news10.com/2015/05/10/skidmore-professor-headed-to-washington-to-talk-about-health/.

Skidmore College. "Diet helps shed pounds, release toxins and reduce oxidative stress." ScienceDaily. ScienceDaily, 11 January 2017. Available at: www.sciencedaily.com/releases/2017/01/170111184102.htm.

"Statistics About Diabetes." American Diabetes Association. Accessed February 23, 2018. http://www.diabetes.org/diabetes-basics/statistics/.

"Stephen F. Austin State University." Kinesiology and Health Science | SFASU. Accessed February 22, 2018. http://www.sfasu.edu/kinesiology.

Streeter, Chris C., Theodore H. Whitfield, Liz Owen, Tasha Rein, Surya K. Karri, Aleksandra Yakhkind, Ruth Perlmutter, Andrew Prescot, Perry F. Renshaw, Domenic A. Ciraulo, and J. Eric Jensen. *Journal of Alternative and Complementary Medicine.* November 2010. Accessed March 20, 2018. https://www.ncbi.nlm.nih.gov/pmc/articles/PMC3111147/.

Taubes, Gary. "What if It's All Been a Big Fat Lie?" *The New York Times.* July 07, 2002. Accessed February 14, 2018. http://www.nytimes.com/2002/07/07/magazine/what-if-it-s-all-been-a-big-fat-lie.html?pagewanted=1.

"The Carnegie Classification of Institutions of Higher Education." Carnegie Classifications | Listings. Accessed January 8, 2018. http://carnegieclassifications.iu.edu/listings.php.

"Try These Four Ways to Slow Down the Ageing Process; Take Control of Your Chronological Age." Coffs Coast Advocate (Coffs Harbour, Australia), February 28, 2015.

Ungar, Peter S., and Mark F. Teaford, eds. *Human Diet: Its Origin and Evolution.* Westport, CT: Bergin and Garvey, 2002.

"US Data & Trends Redirect." Centers for Disease Control and Prevention. April 04, 2012. Accessed February 23, 2018. https://www.cdc.gov/diabetes/statistics/slides/long_ term_trends.pdf .

Valeria, Rosato, Valentina, Maria, Gabriella, Lorenzo, Emilio, Monica, Decarli, and Adriano. "Effect of breakfast composition and energy contribution on cognitive and academic performance: a systematic review | *The American Journal of Clinical Nutrition* | Oxford Academic." OUP Academic. May 27, 2014. Accessed March 8, 2018. https://academic. oup.com/ajcn/article/100/2/626/4576549.

"Vital: 20 FOODS TO BOOST YOUR ENERGY." Daily Record (Glasgow, Scotland), May 17, 2005.

Walford, Roy L. *Beyond the 120-Year Diet: How to Double Your Vital Years.* Revised ed. New York: Four Walls Eight Windows, 2000.

Wang, Duolao, and Ameet Bakhai. *Clinical trials: a practical guide to design, analysis, and reporting.* London: Remedica, 2006.

"Want to Lose Weight? Boost Gut Health for Effective Results." *Hindustan Times* (New Delhi, India), April 23, 2016.

Waterhouse, J., G. Atkinson, B. Edwards, and T. Reilly. "The role of a short post-lunch nap in improving cognitive, motor, and sprint performance in participants with partial sleep deprivation." *Journal of Sports Sciences.* December 2007. Accessed March 15, 2018. https://www.ncbi.nlm.nih.gov/pubmed/17852691.

Weston, Kassia S., Ulrik Wisløff, and Jeff S. Coombes. "High-intensity interval training in patients with lifestyle-induced cardiometabolic disease: a systematic review and meta-analysis." *British Journal of Sports Medicine* 48, no. 16 (2013): 1227-234. doi:10.1136/ bjsports-2013-092576.

"What Is BPA? Should I Be Worried About It?—Mayo Clinic." 2017. Mayo Clinic. http:// www.mayoclinic.org/healthy-lifestyle/nutrition-and-healthy-eating/ expert-answers/ bpa/faq-20058331

Whoriskey, Peter. "The science of skipping breakfast: How government nutritionists may have gotten it wrong." *The Washington Post.* August 10, 2015. Accessed March 18, 2018. https://www.washingtonpost.com/news/wonk/wp/2015/08/10/the-science-of-skipping-breakfast-how-government-nutritionists-may-have-gotten-it-wrong/?utm_ term=.60d3aca497fa.

"Why We Got Fatter During the Fat-Free Food Boom." 2017. NPR.Org. http://www.npr.org/ sections/thesalt/2014/03/28/295332576/ why-we-got-fatter-during-the-fat-free-food-boom

"World Health Organization Assesses the World's Health Systems." WHO. Accessed January 8, 2018. http://www.who.int/whr/2000/media_centre/press_release/en/.

"You Can Now Snort Chocolate, But Doctors Aren't Happy About It." Health.com. Accessed March 10, 2018. http://www.health.com/nutrition/snortable-chocolate-coco-loko.

"Your Health." *Daily Herald* (Arlington Heights, IL), February 13, 2017.

Zohar, Sarah. "Phase I/II Clinical Trials." *Methods and Applications of Statistics in Clinical Trials*, 2014, 658-66. doi:10.1002/9781118596005.ch54.

Zuo, Li, Feng He, Grant M. Tinsley, Benjamin K. Pannell, Emery Ward, and Paul J. Arciero. "Comparison of High-Protein, Intermittent Fasting Low-Calorie Diet and Heart Healthy Diet for Vascular Health of the Obese." *Frontiers in Physiology* 7 (2016). doi:10.3389/fphys.2016.00350.

Appendix A:
Dr. Paul's Protein Pacing Meal Plans

Protein Pacing 1200 Calorie Meal Plan			
	Daily total 30%	Daily total 30%	Daily Total 40%
4 Meals	**Protein, grams**	**Fat, grams**	**Carb, grams**
Breakfast, MMM	23	10	30
Lunch	23	10	30
Dinner	23	10	30
Snack, BBB	23	10	30
Total Grams	92	40	120
5 Meals			
Breakfast, MMM	18	8	24
Morning Snack	18	8	24
Lunch	18	8	24
Dinner	18	8	24
Snack, BBB	18	8	24
Total Grams	90	40	120
6 Meals			
Breakfast, MMM	15	7	20
Morning Snack	15	7	20
Lunch	15	7	20
Afternoon Snack	15	7	20
Dinner	15	7	20
Snack, BBB	15	7	20
Total Grams	90	42	120

Protein Pacing 1500 Calorie Meal Plan			
	Daily total 28%	**Daily total 33%**	**Daily Total 40%**
4 Meals	Protein, grams	Fat, grams	Carb, grams
Breakfast, MMM	27	14	38
Lunch	27	14	38
Dinner	27	14	38
Snack, BBB	27	14	38
Total Grams	108	56	152
5 Meals			
Breakfast, MMM	22	11	30
Morning Snack	22	11	30
Lunch	22	11	30
Dinner	22	11	30
Snack, BBB	22	11	30
Total Grams	110	55	150
6 Meals			
Breakfast, MMM	18	9	25
Morning Snack	18	9	25
Lunch	18	9	25
Afternoon Snack	18	9	25
Dinner	18	9	25
Snack, BBB	18	9	25
Total Grams	108	54	150

Protein Pacing 1800 Calorie Meal Plan			
	Daily total 28%	**Daily total 32%**	**Daily Total 40%**
4 Meals	Protein, grams	Fat, grams	Carb, grams
Breakfast, MMM	32	16	45
Lunch	32	16	45
Dinner	32	16	45
Snack, BBB	32	16	45
Total Grams	128	64	180
5 Meals			
Breakfast, MMM	26	13	36
Morning Snack	26	13	36
Lunch	26	13	36
Dinner	26	13	36
Snack, BBB	26	13	36
Total Grams	130	65	180
6 Meals			
Breakfast, MMM	22	11	30
Morning Snack	22	11	30
Lunch	22	11	30
Afternoon Snack	22	11	30
Dinner	22	11	30
Snack, BBB	22	11	30
Total Grams	132	66	180

Protein Pacing 2000 Calorie Meal Plan			
	Daily total 27%	Daily total 32%	Daily Total 40%
4 Meals	Protein, grams	Fat, grams	Carb, grams
Breakfast, MMM	34	18	50
Lunch	34	18	50
Dinner	34	18	50
Snack, BBB	34	18	50
Total Grams	136	72	200
5 Meals			
Breakfast, MMM	27	14	40
Morning Snack	27	14	40
Lunch	27	14	40
Dinner	27	14	40
Snack, BBB	27	14	40
Total Grams	135	70	200
6 Meals			
Breakfast, MMM	23	12	33
Morning Snack	23	12	33
Lunch	23	12	33
Afternoon Snack	23	12	33
Dinner	23	12	33
Snack, BBB	23	12	33
Total Grams	138	72	198

Protein Pacing 2400 Calorie Meal Plan			
	Daily total 27%	Daily total 36%	Daily Total 40%
4 Meals	Protein, grams	Fat, grams	Carb, grams
Breakfast, MMM	40	24	60
Lunch	40	24	60
Dinner	40	24	60
Snack, BBB	40	24	60
Total Grams	160	96	240
5 Meals			
Breakfast, MMM	32	19	48
Morning Snack	32	19	48
Lunch	32	19	48
Dinner	32	19	48
Snack, BBB	32	19	48
Total Grams	160	95	240
6 Meals			
Breakfast, MMM	27	16	40
Morning Snack	27	16	40
Lunch	27	16	40
Afternoon Snack	27	16	40
Dinner	27	16	40
Snack, BBB	27	16	40
Total Grams	162	96	240

Protein Pacing 3000 Calorie Meal Plan			
	Daily total 25%	Daily total 35%	Daily Total 40%
4 Meals	Protein, grams	Fat, grams	Carb, grams
Breakfast, MMM	45	28	75
Lunch	45	28	75
Dinner	45	28	75
Snack, BBB	45	28	75
Total Grams	180	112	300
5 Meals			
Breakfast, MMM	36	22	60
Morning Snack	36	22	60
Lunch	36	22	60
Dinner	36	22	60
Snack, BBB	36	22	60
Total Grams	180	110	300
6 Meals			
Breakfast, MMM	30	18	50
Morning Snack	30	18	50
Lunch	30	18	50
Afternoon Snack	30	18	50
Dinner	30	18	50
Snack, BBB	30	18	50
Total Grams	180	108	300

Appendix B:
Dr. Paul's PRISE
Intensity Scale for Fitness

INTENSITY LEVEL	DESCRIPTION	EXAMPLE	INTENSITY FACTOR
1	**No Physical Movement**	Seated or standing in a relaxed position.	.1
2	**Very Easy Physical Activity**	Stroll pace or window shopping. Talking is easy and you are not out of breath.	.2
3	**Easy Physical Activity**	A comfortable walk to a destination and able to carry a conversation. You are relaxed and not physically stressed.	.3
4	**Low Physical Activity**	A brisk walk at a pace you can carry a conversation but need to pause occasionally to catch your breath. Your heart is beating quicker and you're breathing a little deeper.	.4
5	**Low-Moderate Physical Activity**	Any activity that increases your heart rate, breathing, and body temperature. You can talk but need to focus on breathing more often with effort. You could maintain this pace for hours, such as during an easy hike.	.5
6	**Moderate Physical Activity**	Moderate-paced activity that starts you sweating, breathing deeper, and increasing your heart rate. You can talk but it takes effort. You could maintain this pace for hours, such as a moderate hike.	.6

7	Moderate-Vigorous Physical Activity	A moderate-vigorous activity that gets you sweating and breathing hard and your heart rate is beating faster. You can only talk during your exhalation. You could maintain this pace up to 2–4 hours, maximum.	.7
8	Vigorous Physical Activity	Faster-paced activity that gets you sweating, breathing hard, and your heart rate is fast. Talking is difficult. You could only maintain for 30–60 minutes, if you really push.	.8
9	Very Vigorous Physical Activity	A near maximum activity effort. You are not able to talk and can only maintain this up to several minutes with your best effort. Unable to talk.	.9
10	"All-out" Burst of Physical Activity	A maximal physical effort, you're breathing as fast as you can, and your heart rate is at its max. You can only maintain this pace up to a minute with full effort. Only grunting and gasping at this level.	1.0

Appendix C:
Dr. Paul's Dynamic Functional Warm-Up Exercises

Before starting each RISE exercise routine, I encourage you to perform a walk/jog warm-up for five minutes at a moderate (Intensity Level 4–7) pace. This should include forward and backward walk/jog/runs of 10–12 yards, repeat for 2 sets.

Following this light walk/jog, I recommend you perform my dynamic warm-up for an additional five to ten minutes using the exercises listed below with some samples shown in picture form. The full exercise warm-up routine can be found in my PRISE App at www.proteinpacing.com, www.priseprotocol.com, and www.paularciero.com.

DYNAMIC WARM-UP:

*For any exercise that requires you to bend your knee, always make sure your knee does not extend over your toes. This will help prevent excessive flexion and stress placed on your knee joint.

Pendulum swings (side-to-side)

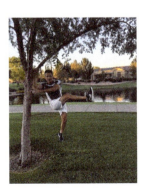
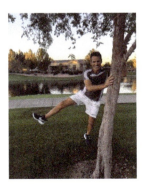

Hold on to a stationary object, freely swing your right leg across your body from right to left while relaxing the muscles in your hip. Increase the range of motion with each swing. Perform 12–15 swings then switch legs. Resist bending at your waist in any direction.

Pendulum swings
(front to back)

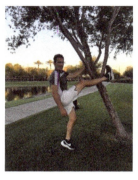 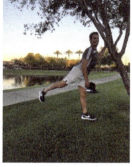

Hold on to stationary object, freely swing leg front to back of your body while relaxing muscles in your hip region. Increase range of motion with each swing. Perform 12–15 swings then switch legs. Try not to bend forward or backward when swinging.

High knee to chest

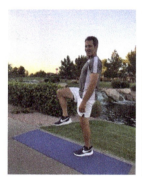 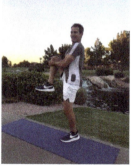

Bend right knee and lift as high as possible, then interlock fingers below knee and lift knee to chest. Keep your back straight and lift onto the ball of your foot. Resist bending forward at the waist. Repeat on left side. Perform 10–12 reps with each leg.

Hip closing

Reach your right knee as far behind you as you can and then lift and bring to the front of your body and place your foot down on the ground. Perform on left side and repeat alternating legs as you go for 12–15 steps forward.

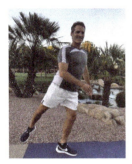 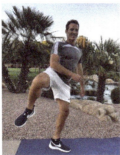 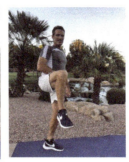 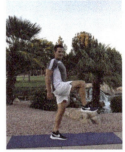

Hip opening

Begin by lifting right knee in front of your body as high as possible then pull back behind your body as you step back. Perform on left side and repeat alternating legs for 12–15 steps backward.

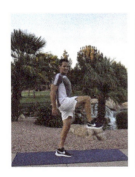 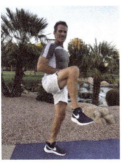 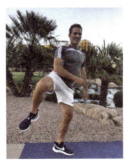 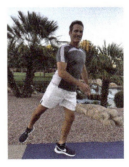

Side shuffle with overhead arm swings

Perform side shuffles while swinging your arms in front of your body down at your waist and overhead. Repeat for 8–10 shuffles then switch directions.

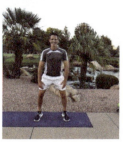 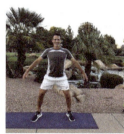 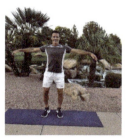 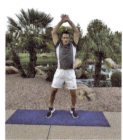

Appendix D:
Dr. Paul's Resistance
Exercise Examples

Side Shuffle with Cones

Place cones ~10 feet apart and side shuffle between cones as quickly as possible, staying low touching each one. Perform continuously for 15–30 seconds and repeat for two sets.

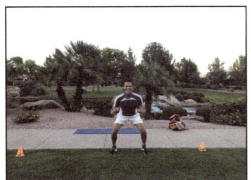 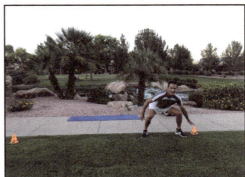

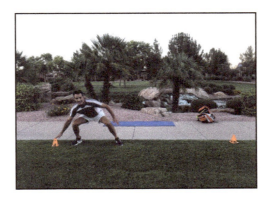

Squats

Place feet about shoulder width apart. Squat down so knees are at 90º and keep hands behind head; come back up to start position. Perform 12–15 reps. Perform 2 sets. Be sure to sit back on your heels so your knees stay behind your toes.

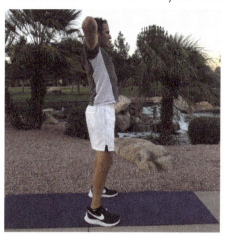
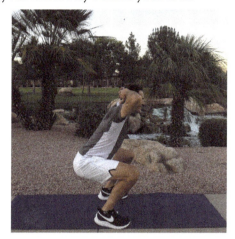

Lunges

Standing with feet hip width apart, step one leg out in a lunge with hands clasped behind your head and then return to standing position. Repeat with each leg 12–15 reps. Perform 2 sets.

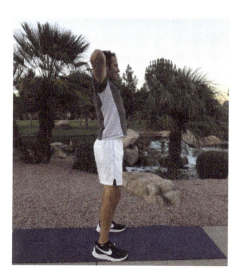
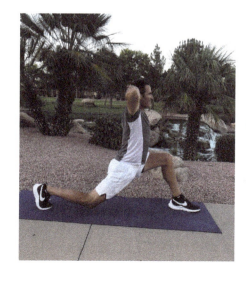

Back Rows

Place band around stationary object. Assume starting position as shown, feet spread apart, tighten core, slightly leaning backward, back straight. Exhale and pull band toward your body alternating among your chest, shoulders, and abdomen. Return to start position. Repeat for 12–15 reps, perform 2 sets.

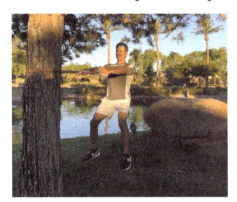 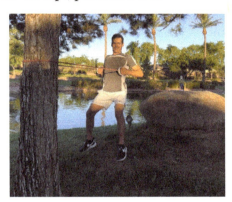

Chest Flies

Place band around stationary object such as a pole, tree, or fence. Grab one handle in each hand and face away from middle of band. Assume start position as shown with arms opened. Tighten core. Bring both hands together in front of your body in a "hug" motion, squeezing your chest muscles together. Vary the height in which you are hugging. For example, alternate among hugging at chest, shoulder, and abdomen height. Slowly return to start position. Perform 12–15 reps and 2 sets.

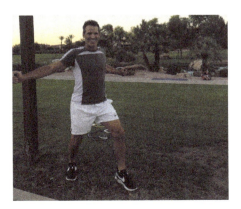 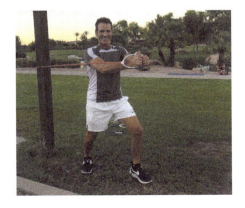

Appendix E:
Dr. Paul's Stretching Exercise Examples

These series of Stretching poses are great for overall muscle flexibility, joint mobility, range of motion, and pliability.

Side Bend Series

Stand with feet together and palms of hands together in front of chest and shoulders relaxed. Exhale and reach both arms overhead. Maintain alignment with spine. Hold for 4 breaths. Slowly lower left arm down your leg and extend your right arm over to your left, reaching as far as you can. Repeat on the right side. Make sure hips remain in alignment. Hold for 4 breaths.

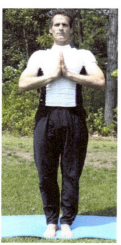 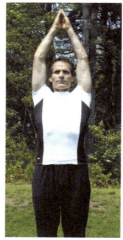 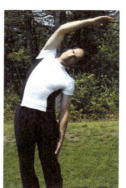 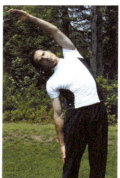

Tree Pose

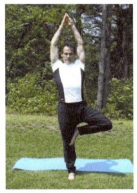 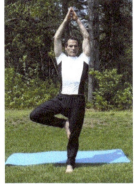

With both arms fully extended overhead, lift your left leg and place the sole of your foot on the inside of your right thigh. Hold this position for 4 breaths and then repeat on the other side.

Forward Bend Series

In standing position with hands in front of chest, slide them down your thighs, holding and exhaling for 4 breaths until you lower your head to your knees. Hold for 4 breaths.

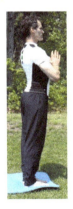 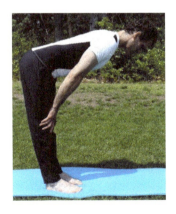 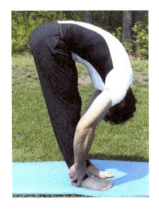

Deep Crescent Stretch

Lower your left knee down to the ground with your right knee bent at 90°. Maintain a straight spine by placing your hands on top of your right thigh. Hold for 4 breaths and repeat on the left side.

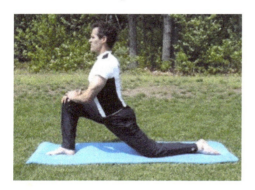
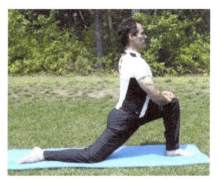

Cat Camel Stretch

Begin with both knees and hands on the ground. Inhale and fully extend your spine by raising your head and dropping your spine to the ground and point your toes. Exhale and flex your spine and curl your toes under your heels. Repeat 4 times.

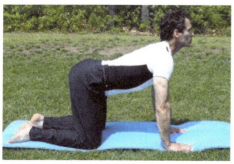
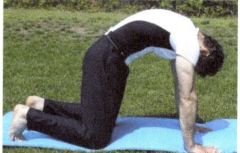

Upward Dog and Child's Pose

Lie on the ground, exhale and push up with your arms until they are fully extended underneath your shoulders; point your toes. Inhale and sit back on your heels and lower your head to the ground. Hold for 4 breaths.

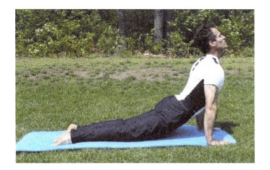

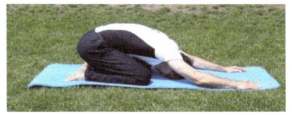

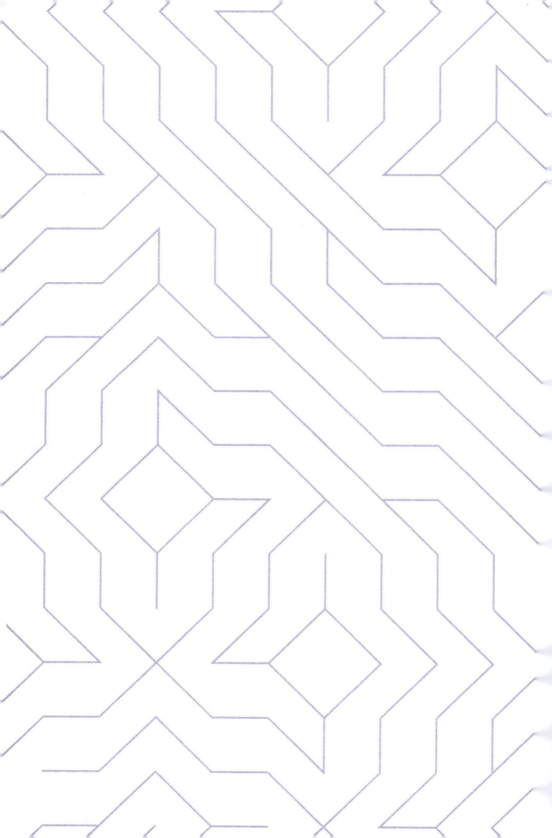

About the Author

Dr. Paul Arciero earned advanced graduate degrees in both Nutrition (Masters of Science) and Applied and Exercise Physiology (Masters of Science, Doctorate, Post-Doctorate Fellowship). He holds advisory board positions of different organizations, including the International Protein Board (iPB, www.internationalproteinboard.com), and is a Fellow of The Obesity Society (FTOS), American College of Sports Medicine (FACSM), and the International Society of Sports Nutrition (FISSN). With over thirty years of dedicated science-based research, he has over fifty-eight peer-reviewed published scientific articles, and is considered a "go-to" content expert by the highest level media outlets, such as O Magazine, The Wall Street Journal, Fox News, Prevention, Good Housekeeping, WebMD, TIME, Huffington Post, Daily Mail, SELF, Glamour, Shape, Health, Women's Health, Women's World, Muscle and Fitness, Men's Fitness, Men's Health, and the list goes well beyond this. He continues to be the "pioneer" and leading expert on teaching how to use Protein Pacing, the PRISE Protocol, and the PRISE App to help you live the "PRISE Life"!

His speeches draw audiences into the tens of thousands, and his devotion to helping people achieve optimal health and peak performance—from Olympians or star athletes to the already overstressed busy person—is contagious.

Join with him to end unhealthy eating and exercise habits worldwide, stop the crazy fad diets and harmful exercise over exertions, and prove that selfcare truly is the new health-care. Do yourself the biggest favor of your life and "Keep your eyes on the PRISE" by never needing to "diet" again! Please visit www.proteinpacing.com, www.paularciero.com and www.priseprotocol.com for more information.

CPSIA information can be obtained
at www.ICGtesting.com
Printed in the USA
LVHW070003071119
636625LV00020B/84/P

9 781478 799474